THE "BIG THREE'S" TAKEOVER OF SPORT

Earle F. Zeigler,
Ph.D., LL.D., D.Sc., FAAKPE
The University of Western Ontario
London, Ontario, Canada

2011

Order this book online at www.trafford.com
or email orders@trafford.com

Most Trafford titles are also available at major online book retailers.

Printed in the United States of America.

ISBN: 978-1-4269-7218-8 (sc)
ISBN: 978-1-4269-7219-5 (e)

Trafford rev. 06/02/2011

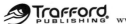

www.trafford.com

North America & International
toll-free: 1 888 232 4444 (USA & Canada)
phone: 250 383 6864 ♦ fax: 812 355 4082

Dedication

I dedicate this book to all those who believe that the finest type of sport competition is connected with the all-important values that, in slightly different forms, are vital for all "valuable" human activities. Among these values are the following:

1. The value of health itself (of course),

2. The value of trying to make a contribution regardless of actual success--the value of effort itself,

3. The value of actual achievement, including excellence,

4. The value of respect for opponents,

5. The value of cooperation (i.e., one's ability to subordinate the self to the attainment of collective goals,

6. The value of fair play (i.e., respect for the rules of competition, which are universalistic ideally),

7. The value of orderly procedure for the settling of disputes, and

8. The value of grace in intensively competitive situations--including magnanimity in victory and the ability to accept defeat gracefully, and then try to gain victory the next time. (

(Note: This listing was developed cooperatively with the late Dr. H. M Johnson, Department of Sociology, University of) Illinois, UIUC

Table of Contents
(and Conceptual Index)

Preface

Some might considered it a no-brainer that an entire book has been written about something that *should* be obvious to just about everyone. However, if it is, that cliché hasn't reached my neighborhood yet. Daily representatives of the media spew out sports stories and incidents in increasing quantity and intensity to the point where even a jaded old–timer such as I has to be careful to keep it all in perspective. There is no mistaking the fact that "big sport" has steadily become a *fourth* powerful social force or influence joining democracy, capitalism, and nationalism in the direction of society in the Western world.

I, the author, was a high school student in America during the years of the "Great Depression" (i.e., the 1930s) after the stock market crash of 1929. Then I worked my way through college in the States. Stepson of a minister, I worked 20-25 hours a week during the school year and full-time summers, for the entire four-year experience. In addition, I played several sports, took part in a variety of campus activities, and had a steady girl friend. Somehow I "survived", but my *formal* education necessarily suffered. Eventually, however, after completing graduate study, working briefly at a YMCA, and following a seven-year experience as physical education instructor and coach at Yale, I became a department head and coached football and also alternated between swimming and wrestling at The U. of Western Ontario in the period from 1949 to 1956. After subsequent administrative and professorial stints at Michigan (Ann Arbor) and Illinois (UIUC), I returned to Western Ontario to become the dean of the new Faculty of Physical Education in 1971. I semi-retired finally in 1989.

I believe strongly that a qualified university student preparing today to contribute to 21st century society should not face the same financial problems as I did. Nevertheless, I am strongly opposed to outright athletic scholarships. I *am* firmly convinced that *all* qualified students with *proven* financial need should be helped in a variety of ways to make their way through the university experience without ending up with a burdensome debt for years to follow.

Keeping my longtime involvement with sport and related physical activity over a period of eighty or so years in mind, I found that I now had no choice but to jump in "media waters" and seek to call a few points to the attention of a seeming gullible public that is saying almost daily: "Aha!

Another sport spectacle to keep us 'sullen, but perhaps not mutinous' as the world continues down its path to a most uncertain future." The general public simply does not understand what has happened: How this "bastardization" of the *true* purpose of competitive sport developed and is continuing "for *worse*, not *better*" to the present!

Yet, just exactly how should I interject myself into this increasingly problematic situation? What a horrendous dilemma it has become! The only logical approach open to me, I now believe, is to simply point out step by step incidences about this or that mistake or inconsistency in society's relationship to sport and related physical activity. As I now see it, after digesting it for myself reluctantly over the years, sport is being used blatantly with unconcern for the results it is creating on varied fronts in society. In addition, as I size it up, the large majority of society is blithely accepting it on the basis of the desires of those—many who are well intentioned—would "use it" that way.

So what we have before us is the social force of democracy "staggering along" as people who would abuse it thrive. This is happening, while those who should use it the democratic system more properly are sitting relatively idly on the sidelines. At the same time ideologues strive to whip healthy patriotism into overwhelming nationalism in a variety of ways now including sport too. Further, subscribers to the "greatness" of economic capitalism either struggle or watch blithely as "the rich get unbelievably richer" in a world where there "may be no tomorrow" worth supporting…

It's not a pretty picture I am painting, this projection averring that the "unholy Big Three" have steadily and increasingly commandeered my longtime, beloved activity known as sport and are "using and abusing" it for their supposedly beneficent purposes.

In this book, then, I'll start by stating what I think many people in the modern world had in mind for sport's purpose. Then I will enumerate in various ways what has happened to what in my youth I blithely thought sport "was all about." Finally, I'll do my best to explain specifically what I think must happen to restore sport to my innocent conception of what the highest aims of competitive sport should be.

Earle F. Zeigler, Richmond, BC, Canada, 2011

Prologue:

This book is titled *The "Big–Three's" Takeover of Sport.* As these words sink in, you may think immediately: "What a great idea?" Conversely, I am arguing here that such a take-over is indeed a most serious problem that gradually became a crisis as the twentieth century wore on. *However, we are now moving along in the twenty-first century!* Thus, if you will bear with me as you get into this book, I believe that you may eventually agree that the "commandeering" of competitive sport by these powerful social forces to serve their avowed purposes is a tragedy of the first magnitude...

Assuming that we are indeed presently being confronted by deep underlying social problems that are having most serious ramifications for our future, what can be done? If such an overall social condition about sport's takeover is true—e.g., that sport is being used by the basic social forces of democracy, capitalism, and nationalism, the "powers that be", it means that we must move to assess the evolving situation more carefully than ever before. O.K., what's wrong with such a development? Isn't the social force of democracy a form of government that is the ideal? It's touted as the best approach for all because *the people* get to rule themselves through the power of the ballot box?

In addition, hasn't capitalism been the social force (i.e., institution) that has shown itself to be the most effective "social engine" to generate business and create a healthy economy in the process. Further, why shouldn't those in control in the leading countries of the Western world using democracy and capitalism be proud and patriotic, even nationalistic in their praise of their countries for having created such a desirable way of life?

Finally, to round off these arguing points, enlightened leaders of these top countries in the West wisely saw that the interest of the people in competitive sport could be harnessed in a variety of ways to solidify everything with an "accompanying layer of competitive sport." Here was an ideal way for the world's countries to help their citizens to build strong pride in their countries' accomplishments. In addition, these ever-growing sport spectacles at all levels were providing a means whereby men and women athletes can compete internationally in sport instead of war. Hence, this a way to create an *ideal* local, provincial, national, and international climate setting an example for the world's countries to emulate?

Well, ladies and gentlemen, I hate to say it, but I'm going to do my best in this book to "rain on your parade–if indeed what I have just described sounds like an ideal arrangement to you. I must report initially that there is now considerable concern "out there" about the way "The Big Three" is doing its job. First, the very large of the people are not getting sufficiently involved so that we can truly say: "Democracy works." Second, capitalism has created a monetary situation where there is a grossly uneven arrangement as to who has the money to purchase life's wherewithal. Third, a desirable level of patriotism throughout the world has too often degenerated into an unhealthy nationalism causing much strife. Finally–and this is the main purpose of this book–the commandeering , or take-over, of sport by the "conglomerate of three" enumerated–has just about created a situation where competitive sport has been increasingly "degraded" to a destructive "professional morality" espousing a mentality that screams: "Winning is not the most important thing in sport; it is the *only* thing!"

To speak to what I see as a real crisis effectively, therefore, I will seek to provide an approach that should help you to understand–and perhaps agree with–what I am saying. However, even if I am successful in convincing you–which I see as most unlikely in the present climate–somehow infusing you with the necessary enthusiasm and vigor that will be required to subsequently communicate with and convince policy makers at all levels about this ever-increasing problem will be almost impossible.

Whatever, at any rate, I decided to use the five–question approach to the building of effective communication skills recommended by Mark Bowden, a communications specialist, to get this effort underway (*National Post*, Canada, 2008 11 24, FP3)

Question 1: Where are we now?

Question 2. Why are we here?

Question 3. Where should we want to be?

Question 4. How do we get there?

Question 5. What exactly should we do?

Without attempting to enumerate specifically where any stumbling blocks might loom in our path, the field of sport management should keep in mind the four major processes proposed by March and Simon (*The Future of Human Resource Management*, 1958, pp. 129-131). They could be employed chronologically, as the field seeks to realize its desired immediate objectives and long-range goal. These four major processes to be followed in the achievement of the desired objectives and goals for the field are as follows:

1. *Problem-solving*: Basically, what is being proposed here is a problem for the profession of sport management to solve or resolve. It must move as soon as possible to convince others that this proposal is truly worthwhile. Part of the approach includes assurance that the objectives are indeed operational (i.e., that their presence or absence can be tested empirically as the field progresses). In this way, even if sufficient funding were not available--and it well might not be--the various parties who are vital or necessary to the success of the venture would at least have agreed-upon objectives. However, with a professional task of this magnitude, it is quite possible, even probable that such consensus will not be achieved initially. *But it can be instituted--one step at a time!*

2. *Persuasion*: For the sake of argument, then, let us assume that the objectives on the way toward the achievement of long-range aims are not shared by the others whom the profession needs to convince, people who are either directly or indirectly related to the field or are in allied fields or related disciplines. On the assumption that the stance of the others is not absolutely fixed or intractable, then this second step of persuasion can (should) be employed on the assumption that at some level our objectives will be shared, and that disagreement over sub-goals can be mediated by reference to larger common goals. (Here the field should keep in mind that influencing specific leaders in each of the various "other" associations and societies with which it is seeking to cooperate can be a most effective technique for bringing about attitude change within the larger membership of our profession everywhere.)

Note: If persuasion works, then the parties concerned can obviously return to the problem-solving level (#1).

3. *Bargaining:* We will now move along to the third stage of a theoretical plan on the assumption that the second step (persuasion) didn't fully work. This means obviously that there is still disagreement over the operational goals proposed at the problem-solving level (the first stage). Now the field has a difficult decision to make: does it attempt to strike a bargain, or do it decide that we simply must "go it alone?"

The problem with the first alternative is that bargaining implies compromise, and compromise means that each group involved will have to surrender a portion of its claim, request, or argument. The second alternative may seem more desirable, but following it may also mean eventual failure in achieving the final, most important objective.

Note: We can appreciate, of course, that the necessity of proceeding to this stage, and then selecting either of the two alternatives, is obviously much less desirable than settling the matter at either the first or second stages.

4. *Politicking:* The implementation of the fourth stage (or plan of attack) is based on the fact that the proposed action of the first three stages has failed. The participants in the discussion cannot agree in any way about the main issue. It is at this point that the recognized profession of sport management has to somehow expand the number of parties or groups involved in consideration of the proposed project. The goal, of course, is to attempt to include potential allies so as to improve the chance of achieving the desired final objective. Employing so-called "power politics" is usually tricky, however, and it may indeed backfire upon the group bringing such a maneuver into play.

However, this is the way the world (or society) works, and the goal may be well worth the risk or danger involved.

> Note: Obviously, the hope that it will not be necessary to operate at this fourth stage continually in connection with the development of the field. It would be most divisive in many instances and time consuming as well. Therefore, the field would be faced with the decision as to whether this type of operation would do more harm than good (in the immediate future at least).

PART ONE: WHERE ARE WE NOW?

Chapter 1
Sport As a Key Partner
in the
"Big Four's Reign"

Sport has obviously become an extremely powerful social force in society. If we grant that it now has such power in our culture—a power indeed that appears to be growing steadily—we can also recognize that any such social force affecting society can be dangerous if perverted (e.g., positive nationalism to blind chauvinism; normal commercialism to excessive commercialism; wholesome sport competition to "own-the-podium mentality"). Assuming the rationale behind these assertions, I believe that, while sport has grown as an important social force, it now also appears to have become a societal institution with an inadequately defined theory.

Within this presently muddled situation in regard to sport's role in society, I feel that most people—including the writer as a person concerned with the social-science and philosophic aspects of sport—are like the proverbial blind person attempting to describe an elephant using the sense of touch only (i.e., here a trunk, there a tusk, next four leathery pillars, etc.). Even though we humans have sight, we are akin to a person attempting to assemble a jigsaw puzzle without first seeing the complete picture on the cover of the box. This had led us into developing warped or truncated ideas about the big picture of sport we should be assembling in a presumably forward-looking society. Resultantly, this causes us to ignore concomitant benefits attained from participation in, or observance of, competitive sport activities, as well as in more basic exercise and expressive movement.

The "big four" named in the title of this brief statement are "ruling" the Western world. **First,** *Democracy* is promoted vigorously as the most desirable type of political institution. **Second**, *economic capitalism* is being promoted as the most worthwhile social institution, albeit with certain reservations by a significant minority. **Third**, *nationalism* is promulgated as important "love of country" vital for a country's development in an uncertain world. Now, **fourth**, and most interestingly, *competitive sport* during the 20th century somehow has also become *a fourth important social institution* promulgated to serve the "best interests" of humanity. The implication is, of course, that democracy, capitalism, nationalism, and sport should continue to function as is and even brought to play vigorously in the twenty-first century. It is evidently believed that each "force" singly will bring about more "good" than "bad." Finally, the ongoing contribution of each to the collective whole will lead to "a good future" for humankind on earth. (How this will play out for so-called "third–world" countries will be a theme for another day…)

However, in each case, we are finding this assumption that "all's well" is being challenged. In America, for example, only half of the people eligible to vote in the major election do so, and only one in three votes in the off-year election. The top officials are acting increasingly as "czars." In some countries, therefore, they seem blocked or paralyzed and are not functioning well. Somehow, although all citizens "have the vote" and could potentially "be involved" positively, things aren't heading in that direction. At the same time, in the United States, for example, in the year 2000, there were 791,600 *black* men in *prison* and 603,032 enrolled in colleges and universities. As of June 30, 2008, there are 846,000 *black male* inmates held in state or federal prisons. Let's face it; in addition, the gap between the rich and the poor is increasing at a most alarming rate.

What will this mean as we move along in the 21st century? Will capitalism be made more "palatable" by adding just enough "socialism" so that we can claim with certainty that the "total package" will produce more "good" than "bad"? If you saw Michael Moore's startling 2009 film titled "Capitalism: A Love Story," you'll be hard pressed to believe that we can bank on it…

Division #3 of the "Big Four's reign" is nationalism. Whereas patriotism might refer to "love of country," nationalism could be considered as the blending of patriotism with an accompanying consciousness of nationality. It is a political philosophy in which the good of the nation is supreme, thus leading to an almost unbridled state at its extreme. The word "nationalism" itself might apply to a feeling, attitude, or consciousness that persons might have as citizens of a nation-citizens who hold a strong attitude about the welfare of their nation, about its status in regard to strength or prosperity. Thus defined, nationalism (the third social force discussed briefly here) has been evident throughout the history of civilization from the relatively simple organization of the tribe to the complex nation-states of the modern world. Statesmen and politicians have been quick to seize upon presumed love of country to "drag people along" to do things that "in the light of day," they subsequently regret. However, this does appear to be exactly what is happening today as nationalism is "merged" or "meshed" with the social forces described as democracy and capitalism.

The fourth division of the "Big Four's reign" in North America especially is here designated as "commercialized sport." The development of what has now become a social institution involving highly competitive sport, for example, has reached the point where a claim can be made that it may be doing more harm than good—albeit that such involvement soundly enhances the effort of economic capitalism within the "Big Four." Oddly, the totality of the Western world seemingly has no awareness of this contention and permits sport's ongoing expansion without question. The conventional wisdom appears to be: "Commercialized sport is good for people, and the more spectator involvement there is with it the better." (Shades of Ancient Rome…)

Conversely, and concurrently, the large majority of the population in the so-called developed world is getting *inadequate* involvement in developmental and recreational *physical* activity. Resultantly, it has even been argued recently that the coming generation will be the first to die before their parents. Obesity "reigns" at all periods of life! And yet the truth is that we who function in the field of physical activity education (and related health education) know that—well taught!—such involvement can be a wonderful, health-producing, educational and/or recreational experience for a young person. Hence, we can only *recommend strongly* that all boys and girls should have a required, regular, excellent, graduated program—including related health & safety education. This overall program should include intramural sport competition up to high school graduation.

As it has developed, the problem is that the United States (and Canada too) as democratic countries have typically "got it backwards." Whatever "bona fide," educational/recreational experiences are "out there" are *not* typically made available to ALL children and youth. Hence we must *demand* that those experiences deemed essential for "the finest life" in a democracy be mandated regularly up through high school graduation for all to the extent that each person is capable of being involved. In addition, fully qualified, full-time teacher/coaches should be available to provide these educational experiences.

When these curriculum needs are met, if funding can be made

available, **ALL** children and youth should be able to choose to get involved with **EXTRA-CURRICULAR OPPORTUNITIES** in (1) physical, as well as in (2) social, (3) communicative, (4) aesthetic & creative, and (5) "learning" recreational interests. Whether these opportunities are made available through public education **OR** public recreation should make no difference theoretically.

We can grant that some parents are in a position financially to provide additional experiences for their offspring. Additionally, if "government" chooses to get involved to a reasonable extent in the promotion of any of these educational and recreational experiences for youth, that's fine too. However, it must be understood that such should occur *only if* the *basic* curriculum needs listed above–for all have been met!!! "**EXCELLENCE**" should be the goal in *extramural* or *varsity* sport, but it should come "from the ground-up", *not* from a "top-down, own the podium, subsidizing mentality" anxious to prove that **"WE ARE THE GREATEST!"**.

Further, it is ironic that almost all of the others in the "under-privileged" nations of the world are typically getting too much physical labor and accompanying inadequate, unhealthy nourishment. In addition, these "first world" people are ironically being urged daily to pay increasing amounts of money to watch "skilled others" play competitive games.

The basic problem here in the words of the eminent sport philosopher, Robert G. Osterhoudt, is that "we are fashioning an *instrumental* view of sport, a view that misses sport's basically human (its intrinsic) merits, and thus likewise misses the significance of providing the experience of authentic sport to all people (men and women, young and old, rich and poor) in all nations." Only in such terms may sport justifiably claim itself essential to a good life and as such justifiably claim itself promoting the good of each and all. The world must figure out the ways and means of avoiding the current, zany excesses of "First-World cultures" and the unacceptable deprivations of those cultures designated as "Third-World."

In conclusion, I am forced to ask "*Exactly what is it that we are promoting, and why are we doing it?*" Frankly, I greatly fear the answer. Maybe it's my age, but, frankly, I am "running scared"! It can be argued that this plight has developed because we haven't created a theory of developmental physical activity including sport that permits us to assess whether sport, for example, is fulfilling its presumed function of promoting good in a society. In addition, why do most sport philosophy and social-science scholars assiduously avoid scholarly consideration of exercise and dance as part of their domain? At present these scholars tend definitely to be elitist with their "heads in the sand." Wittingly, or unwittingly, they are seemingly playing ball with and abetting the forces of the "Big Four" explained above.

In addition, I ask the members of the North American Society for Sport Management—and indirectly all other people who hold memberships in similar sport management societies worldwide—what are you and your society doing to cause sport to serve society as a worthwhile social force? From my perspective I can only report that I have seen far too much interest in the promotion of highly organized, commercialized sport for ticket-buying spectators—and far too little—if any!—interest in the promotion of healthful, recreational sport and related physical activity for the very large majority of normal and special-population people of all ages.

I can only conclude that sport is not serving society anywhere well nearly as well as it might... Prove me wrong in the years ahead...

Chapter 2
Sport's Role in the Postmodern World

Characterizations of Competitive Sport

Having stated that "sport" has become a strong social institution, it is true also that there has been some ambiguity about what such a simple word as sport means. The word "sport" is used in many different ways as a noun. The number of definitions is now 14 in the *Encarta World English Dictionary* (1999, p. 1730). In essence, what is being described here in this book is an athletic activity requiring skill or physical prowess. It is typically of a competitive nature as in racing, wrestling, baseball, tennis, or cricket. For the people involved, sport is often serious, and participants may even advance to a stage where competitive sport becomes a career choice as either a semiprofessional or a professional athlete. For most others, however, sport is seen more as a diversion, recreational in nature, and a pleasant pastime.

A Social Institution Without a Theory.

Viewed collectively, my argument here is that at present the "totality" of sport appears to have become a strong social institution--but one that is without a well-defined theory. This assertion may have been recognized by others too. Yet, at this point the general public, including most politicians, seems to believe that "the more competitive sport we have, the merrier!" However, those who seek to promote sport ought right now to be able to answer such questions as (1) what purposes competitive sport has served in the past, (2) what functions it is fulfilling now, (3) where it seems to be heading, and (4) how it should be employed to serve all humankind.

How Sport Serves Society .

In response to these questions, without careful delineation or any priority at this point, I can state that sport as presently operative can be subsumed in a non-inclusive list as possibly serving in the following ways:

> 1. As an organized religion (for those with or
> without another similar competing affiliation)
>
> 2. As an exercise medium (often a sporadic one)
>
> 3. As a life-enhancer or "arouser" (puts

excitement in life)

4. As a trade or profession (depending upon
one's involvement with it)

5. As an avocation, perhaps as a "leisure-filler"
(at either a passive, vicarious, or active level)

6. As a training ground for war (used throughout
history for this purpose)

7. As a "socializing activity" (an activity where
one can meet and enjoy friends)

8. As an educational means (i.e., the development
of positive character traits, however described)

In retrospect, I find it most interesting that I didn't list sport "as
a developer of positive character traits" until last! Now I wonder
why. . . .

This listing could undoubtedly be larger. It could have included such
terms as (1) sport "the destroyer," (2) sport "the redeemer," (3) sport "the
social institution being tempted by science and technology," (4) sport "the
social phenomenon by which heroes and villains are created," or, finally, (5)
sport "the social institution that has survived within an era characterized by
a vacuum of belief for many." However, I must stop. believing this listing is
sufficient to make the necessary point here.

The hope is that you, the reader, will agree that those people involved
in the sport enterprise truly need to understand what competitive sport has
become in society. Frankly, I don't believe that a great many of its promoters
know they are confronted with a stark dilemma. My argument here is that
sport too--as is true for all other social institutions--will inevitably be
confronted by the postmodern divide. In crossing this frontier, many
troubling and difficult decisions, often ethical in nature, will have to be made
by those related to commercialized sport in one of several ways. For
example, what sort of professional preparation should prospective sport
managers and coaches have, those men and women who will guide sport
into becoming a responsible social institution? The fundamental question

facing the profession is: "What kind of sport does this presently "amorphous enterprise" seek to promote to help shape what sort of world we will be living in for the rest of the 21st century?"

Is Sport Fulfilling Its Presumed Educational and Recreational Roles Adequately?

Specifically, what implications arise from this dilemma for sport? As I view it, there are strong indications that sport's presumed educational and recreational roles in the "adventure" of civilization are not being fulfilled adequately. Frankly, the way commercialized, overemphasized sport has been operated, I believe it can be added to the list of symptoms of American internal decay enumerated above (e.g., drugs, violence, decline of intellectual interest, dishonesty, greed). If true, this inadequacy inevitably throws a burden on sport management as a profession to try to do something about it. Sport, along with all of humankind, is simply facing the postmodern divide.

Reviewing this claim in some detail, Depauw (Quest, 1997) argues that society should demonstrate more concern for those who have traditionally been marginalized in society by the sport establishment (i.e., those excluded because of sex or "physicality"). She speaks of "The (In)Visibility of DisAbility" in our culture. Depauw's position is backed substantively by what Blinde and McCallister (1999) call "The Intersection of Gender and Disability Dynamics."

A second point of contention about sport's contribution relates to the actual "sport experience." The way much sport has been conducted, the public has every right to ask, "Does sport build character or 'characters'?" Kavussannu & Roberts (2001) recently showed that, even though "sport participation is widely regarded as an important opportunity for character development," it is also true that sport "occurs in a context that values ego orientation (e.g. winning IS the most important thing)."

Sport's Contribution Today

What is competitive sport's contribution today? Delving into this matter might produce a surprise, or perhaps not. It may well be that sport is contributing significantly in the development of what are regarded as instrumental, social values (i.e., the values of teamwork, loyalty, self-sacrifice, and perseverance consonant with prevailing corporate capitalism in democracy and other political systems as well. Conversely, however, there is now growing evidence that sport is developing an ideal that opposes the fundamental moral virtues of honesty, fairness, and responsibility in the innumerable competitive experiences provided (Lumpkin, Stoll, and Beller, 1999).

Significant to this discussion are the results of investigations carried out by Hahm, Stoll, Beller, Rudd, and others in the late 1980s and 1990s. The Hahm-Beller Choice Inventory (HBVCI) has now been administered to athletes at different levels in a variety of venues. It demonstrates conclusively that athletes will not support what is considered "the moral ideal" in competition. As the argument goes, an athlete with moral character should demonstrate the moral character traits of honesty, fair play, respect, and responsibility whether an official is present to enforce the rules or not. This finding was substantiated by Priest, Krause, and Beach (1999), They reported that their findings in the four-year changes occurring in college athletes' ethical value choices were consistent with other investigations. This study a;so showed decreases in "sportsmanship orientation" and an increase in "professional" attitudes associated with sport.

On the other hand, even though dictionaries define social character similarly, sport practitioners, including participants, coaches, parents, and officials, have come to believe that character is defined properly by such values as self-sacrifice, teamwork, loyalty, and perseverance (Rudd, et al., 1999). The common expression in competitive sport is: "He/she showed character"-meaning "He/she 'hung in there' to the bitter end!" [or whatever]. Rudd confirmed also that coaches explained character as "work ethic and commitment." This coincides with what sport sociologists have found, also, Sage (1988, p. 634) explained that "Mottoes and slogans such as 'sports builds character' must be seen in the light of their ideological issues" In other words, competitive sport is typically structured by the nature of the society in which it occurs. This would appear to mean that over-commercialization, drug-taking, cheating, bribe-taking by officials, violence, etc. at all levels of sport are simply reflections of the culture in which we live.

Thus, we are left with sport's presumed relationship with moral character development that has been misinterpreted. And so, despite its early 20th-century claims to be "the last best hope on earth" for immigrants, American culture--where this "redefinition" of the term character has occurred--appears to be facing what Berman (2000) calls "spiritual death" (p.

52). He makes this claim because of "its crumbling school systems and widespread functional illiteracy, violent crime and gross economic inequality, and apathy and cynicism."

At this point, one can't help but recall that the ancient Olympic Games became so excessive with ills that the event was abolished. The Games were begun again only by the spark provided in the late 19th century by Baron de Coubertin's "noble amateur ideal." The way things are going today, it is not unthinkable that the steadily increasing excesses of the present Olympic Games Movement could well bring about its demise again. However, they could well be only symptomatic of a larger problem confronting world culture.

This discussion about whether sport's presumed educational and recreational roles have justification in fact could go on indefinitely. So many negative incidents have occurred that one hardly knows where to turn to avoid further negative examples. On the one hand we read the almost unbelievably high standards set in the Code of Conduct developed by the Coaches Council of the National Association for Sport and Physical Education (NASPE, 2001). Conversely, however, we learn that today athletes' concern for the presence of moral values in sport declines over the course of a university career (Priest, Krause, and Beach, 1999).

Sedentary Living Has Caught Up With America.

With this as a backdrop, we learn further that Americans are, for example, concurrently increasingly facing the cost and consequences of sedentary living (Booth & Chakravarthy, 2002). Additionally, Malina (2001) tells us there is a need to track people's physical activity across their life spans. North America hasn't yet been able to devise and accept a uniform definition of wellness for all people. The one thought that emerges from these various assessments is as follows: Many people give every evidence of wanting their "sport spectaculars" for the few--much more than they want all people of all ages and all conditions to have meaningful sport, exercise, and physical recreation involvements throughout their lives!

In Canada, conversely, Tibbetts (2002), for example, described a most recent Environics survey that explained that "65% of Canadians would like more government money spent on local arenas, playgrounds, and swimming pools, as well as on sports for women, the poor, the disabled, and aboriginals." This is not to argue that Canada does not face problems of its own in this area (e.g., professional hockey).

Official Sport's Response to the Prevailing Situation

How does what is often called the "sport officialdom" respond to this situation? Answers to this question are just about everywhere as we think, for example, of the various types of scandals tied to both the summer and winter versions of the Olympic Games. For example, the Vancouver Province (2000) reported that the former "drug czar" of the U.S.A. Olympic Team, Dr. Wade Exum, charged that half of the team used performance-enhancing drugs to prepare for the 1996 Games. After making this statement, the response was rapid: he was forced to resign! He then sued the United States Olympic Committee for racial discrimination and harassment.

Viewed in a different perspective, as reported by Wallis (2002), Dr. Vince Zuaro, a longtime rules interpreter for Olympic wrestling, said recently: "Sports are so politica!. If you think what happened with Enron is political, [try] Olympic officiating. . . Every time there's judging involved, there's going to be a payoff." Further, writing about the credibility of the International Olympic Committee, Feschuk (2002) stated in an article titled "Night of the Olympic Dead": "The IOC has for so long been inflicting upon itself such severe ethical trauma that its survival can only be explained by the fact that it has passed over into the undead. Its lifeless members shuffle across the globe in a zombie-like stupor, one hand extended to receive gratuities, the other held up in exaggerated outrage to deny any accusations of corruption."

At the same time, Dr. Ayotte, director of the only International Olympic Committee-accredited testing laboratory in Canada, explained that young athletes have come believe they must take drugs to compete successfully. "People have no faith in hard work and food now," she says, to achieve success in sport (Long, 2001).

Dick Pound's Reward for Distinguished Service.

Closing out reference to the Olympic Games Movement, recall the case of Dick Pound, the Canadian lawyer from Montreal, who had faithfully, intelligently, and loyally striven most successfully to bolster the Games' finances in recent decades. He had also taken on the assignment of monitoring the situation with drugs and doping, as well as the bribery scandal associated with the Games held in Salt Lake City. In the election to succeed retiring President Samaranch, Pound unbelievably finished in third place immediately behind a man caught in a bribery scandal just a short time earlier (and since removed from office).

Finally, in the realm of international sport, Dr. Hans B. Skaset (2002), a Norwegian professor, in response to a query about a prediction he made at a conference on drugs in sport in November, 2002 e-mailed me a statement he made as a conference keynote speaker:

> Top international sport will cut itself free from its historical values and norms. After working with a clear moral basis for many years, sport by 2008-2010 will continue to be accepted as a leading genre within popular culture--but not, as it was formerly, a model for health, fairness, and honorable conduct. . . .

Switching venues back to North America, you don't see hockey promoters doing anything to really curb the Neanderthal antics of professional hockey players. Considering professional sport generally, also, note the view of sport sociologist, Steven Ortiz, who has found in his study that "there clearly seems to be a 'fast-food sex' mentality among professional athletes" (Cryderman, 2001).

In addition, in the realm of higher education, Canadian universities are gradually moving toward the athletic-scholarship approach that certain universities in the East and Midwest sections of Canada have been following illegally for years (Naylor, 2002)! In September, 2001, a Halifax, Nova Scotia university team, the St. Mary Huskies, beat Mount Allison, a Sackville, New Brunswick university football team in the same conference, by a score of 105-0. In this article, one of a series sponsored by The Globe and Mail (Toronto), various aspects of this lopsided development were considered. Interestingly, funding for recruited athletes is just "penny-ante" compared to the support provided for the scholarship programs of various upper-division

How to Reclaim Sport (Weiner)

In writing about how society's obsession with sport has "ruined the game," Weiner (2000), an insightful sport critic with the Minneapolis Star-Tribune, asked the question: "How far back must we go to remember that sports matter?" Recalling the time when "sports had meaning," and "sports were accessible," he recommends that society can only "reclaim sports from the corporate entertainment behemoth" if it does the following:

1. De-professionalize college and high school sports,
2. Allow some form of public ownership of professional sports teams,
3. Make sports affordable again, and
4. Be conscious of the message sport is sending.

To summarize, it is evident that the leaders of the "sport industry" have quite simply been conducting themselves in keeping with the prevailing political environment and ethos of the general public. They have presumably not understood, and accordingly not accepted, the contention that there is an urgent need for sport to serve as a beneficent social institution with an underlying theory looking to humankind's betterment (a necessary "if 'this,' then 'that' will result" type of approach).

Of course, it can be argued that society does indeed believe that competitive sport is doing what it is intended to do--i.e., provide both non-moral and moral values to those involved in one way or another. (The non-moral values could be listed as recognition, money, and a certain type of power, whereas the moral values could be of a nature designed to help the team achieve victory--dedication, loyalty, self-sacrifice.) If this assessment is accurate, the following question must be asked: Does the prevailing ethos in sport competition need to be altered so that this activity truly helps boys and girls, and men and women too, to learn honesty fair play, justice, responsibility, and beneficence (i.e., doing good)?

Seemingly the only conclusion to be drawn today is that the sport industry is "charging ahead" driven by the prevailing capitalistic, "global village" image of the future. Increasingly in competitive sport, such theory is embraced ever more strongly, an approach in which winning is overemphasized with resulting higher profits to the promoters through increased gate receipts. This same sport industry is aided and abetted by a society in which the majority do not recognize sufficiently the need for sport to serve as a social institution that results in a substantive amount of individual and social good. On the one hand there are scholars who argue that democratic states, under girded by the various human rights legislated (e.g., equal opportunity), urgently need a supportive "liberal consensus" to maintain a social system that is fair to all. Yet, conservative, essentialist elements functioning in the same social system evidently do not see this need for a more humanistic, pragmatic consensus about the steadily mounting evidence showing a need for ALL people to be active physically throughout their lives.

This is the substantive aspect of the basis for the argument that commercialized sport will have great difficulty "crossing the postmodern divide." Zeigler (1996b) pointed out that almost every approach to "the good life" stresses a need for an individual's relationship to developmental physical activity such as sport and fitness. Question: Should not governments and professional associations worldwide be assessing the social institution of sport to determine whether the way sport is presented to students and young people is resulting in their becoming imbued with a desire to promote the concept of "sport for all" to foster overall human betterment?

Functioning With an Indeterminate, Muddled Theory

Before considering future societal scenarios that world culture is facing, the argument should be made again that today sport is functioning vigorously with an indeterminate, muddled theory implying that sport competition builds both "moral" and "social-instrumental" character traits consonant with democracy and capitalism. Crossing the postmodern divide means basically also that sport management educators, for example, should see through the false front and chicanery of the developing economic and technological facade of the global hegemony being promoted. They should be certain that their students understand this shaky development as it might affect their future. Face it: Sport is simply being promoted because it is indeed a powerful institution in this "Brave New World" of the 21st century.

Crossing the Postmodern Divide

Whether we all recognize it or not, similar to all other professions today, the burgeoning sport management profession conceivable may be facing (i.e., striving to cross what has been termed the postmodern divide) An epoch in civilization approaches closure when many of the fundamental convictions of its advocates are challenged by a substantive minority of the populace. It can be argued that indeed the world is moving into a new epoch as the proponents of postmodernism have been affirming over recent decades. Within such a milieu there are strong indications that sport management is going to have great difficulty crossing this chasm, this so-called, postmodern divide.

A diverse group of postmodern scholars argues that many in democracies, under girded by the various rights being propounded (e.g., individual freedom, privacy), have come to believe that now they too require--and deserve!--a supportive "liberal consensus" within their respective societies. Conservative, essentialist elements prevail at present and are functioning strongly in many Western political systems. With their more authoritative orientation in mind, conservatives believe the deeper foundation justifying this claim of a need for a more liberal consensus has never been fully rationalized. However, it can be argued that postmodernists now form a substantive minority supporting a more humanistic, pragmatic, liberal consensus in which present highly competitive sport is viewed as an increasingly negative influence on society (Borgman, 1993, p. 78). If this statement has merit, there are strong indications that the present sport management profession- as known today will have difficulty crossing this postmodern divide that has been postulated.

PART II: HOW DID WE GET HERE?

Chapter 3
Excess in Commercialized Sport Is Threatens Sport's Potential Value to Humankind!

Humankind's struggle to "make a go of it" in the 20th century starkly outlines what now confronts humanity in the 21st century. Living together peacefully, of course, is an ever-present challenge of the highest magnitude. The great historian, Toynbee, reminded us that civilizations died when they simply did not confront challenges successfully. Climate change, for example, is rapidly developing into such a challenge, as are the ongoing clashes of unwavering essentialistic religions.

There is another challenge, however, that the world's populace does not seem to recognize that it has. I am referring to human involvement with sport characterized increasingly by overemphasis, commercialism, and violence as it "progresses professionally, technologically, and commercially." This now appears to have reached the point that it may be having a negative influence on society overall, as well as on the quality and quantity of sport and physical activity programs of children and youth.

Technology and Life Improvement.

Leo Marx (1990, p. 3) asked cogently earlier whether improved technology actually means progress when he stated:

> "Conspicuous disasters have helped to undermine the public's faith in progress, but there has also been a longer-term change in our thinking. . . . Our very conception--our chief criterion—of progress has undergone a subtle but decisive change since the founding of the Republic, and that change is at once a cause and a reflection of our current disenchantment with technology." (p. 5)

"Confusion still prevails" as to whether developing technology is good for society or not! The answer seems to be "yes" and "no". How did humankind create such a dilemma for itself?

It appears that we must look backwards before we can look forwards on the topic. The factory system with its improved machinery that was developing initially in the West in the late 18th century meshed with the thought that history would display "onward and upward" progress. This idea came to dominate American thought and correlated with "Enlightenment thought" emanating from Europe. Science and technology had become partners and resultantly all aspects of life would improve steadily.

Recall that there were two worldviews in the West: the Liberal and the Conservative. Thomas Jefferson in America and like-minded theorists were classical liberals. Jefferson, a political philosopher, was fully imbued with the spirit of the Enlightenment and knew many intellectual leaders in Britain and France. Classical Liberals believed in the right of individuals to control their economic destinies through capitalism, a position in conflict with the Conservative who wished to conserve the values inherited from European traditions.

However, by 1850 the idea of progress was already being separated from the Enlightenment vision of political liberation. "This dissociation of technological and material advancement from the larger political vision of progress was an intermediate stage in the eventual impoverishment of that radical eighteenth-century worldview" (Marx, p. 9). By the turn of the 20th century, the steady material development of the 19th century resulted in "the technocratic idea of progress [becoming] a belief in the sufficiency of scientific and technological innovation as the basis for general progress" (p. 9). This soon came to mean that if scientific-based technologies were permitted to develop in an unconstrained manner, there would be an automatic improvement in all other aspects of life! Thus, Marx argues, that "the Jeffersonian ideal [was turned] on its head, this view making instrumental values fundamental to social progress, and relegating what formerly were considered primary, goal-setting values (justice, freedom, harmony, beauty, or self-fulfillment) to a secondary state" (p. 9).

The "original faith" did not die, however; it lived on in a variety of political thrusts: utopian socialism, the populist revolt, progressivism in cities, the single-tax movement, and Marxism with its many variants. Hence, the "battle was on" during the 20th century between those encouraging spiraling technological advancements and those relatively few intellectuals who could see its inherent dangers most vividly. "This moral critique of the debased, technocratic version of the progressive worldview has slowly gained adherence since the mid-nineteenth century, and by now it is one of the chief ideological supports of an adversary culture in the United States" (p. 12).

Because of this tremendous material progress in the first half of the 20th century, people arguing this way were typically viewed as impractical intellectuals, hopelessly idealistic, etc. Starting in the 1960s, however, and continuing during the last quarter of the 20th century and into the 21st century, there has been a distinct growth of skepticism and a concurrent stronger adversary culture that has gained definite intellectual respect.

The basic question appears, therefore, to be: Are these scientific and technological advancements *MEANS* to an end, or simply *ENDS* in themselves? If improved technology means progress, evidently the leading ideological position today, the next question is--"Progress toward what?" So the fundamental question still today is, "which type of values will win out in the long run?" In North America, for example, it seems that a gradually prevailing concept of cultural relativism was increasingly discredited as the 1990s witnessed a sharp clash between (1) those who uphold so-called Western cultural values and (2) those who by their presence are dividing the West along a multitude of ethnic and racial lines. This is occasioning strong efforts to promote religions and sects based on fundamental beliefs–either those present historically or those recently imported–characterized typically by decisive right/wrong morality.

Agreement on the point that the world has indeed come to rely on science and accompanying technology, we should understand nevertheless that equating technology with progress depends on how one defines the term "progress". However conceived, there can be no argument but that the world faces a variety of extremely threatening challenges in the 21st century.

An Unrecognized Challenge to Modern Society

Keeping what has been written to this point in mind, I believe there is one challenge that the world's populace does not seem to recognize that it has. I am referring to the type of human involvement with sport that is characterized increasingly by overemphasis, commercialism, and violence as sport "progresses" professionally, technologically, and commercially. In my opinion, such involvement now appears to have reached the point that it may be having more of a negative influence on society overall than a positive one. This opinion extends as well from that of so-called elite sport to the quality and quantity of sport and physical activity programs of children, youth, and adults, including those with special needs.

Competitive sport and related physical activity has gradually, but steadily, become a social institution that surged to an extremely powerful social force in the 20th century. I have been attempting to analyze it philosophically and sociologically as to the "use" and "possible abuse" of sport. The underlying theoretical argument is that society is governed by strong social institutions (i.e., "forces"). Among those social institutions are (1) the values (including created norms based on these values), (2) the type of political state in vogue, (3) the prevailing economic system, (4) the religious beliefs present, etc. To these longstanding institutions, I have added the influence of such others as education, the communication media, science. and technological advancement, concern for peace, and now sport itself. (Zeigler, 2003, p. 74). Of all of these, the values a society holds, and the accompanying norms developed on the basis of these values, form the strongest institution of all!

Humankind's struggle to "make a go of it" in the 20th century starkly outlined what now confronts humanity in the 21st century. Living together peacefully, of course, is an ever-present challenge of the highest magnitude. The great historian, Toynbee, reminded us that civilizations died when they simply did not confront challenges successfully. Climate change, for example, is rapidly developing into such a challenge, as are the ongoing clashes of unwavering religions.

There is another challenge, however, that the world's populace does not seem to recognize that it has. I am referring to human involvement with sport characterized increasingly by overemphasis, commercialism, and violence as it "progresses professionally, technologically, and commercially." This now appears to have reached the point that it may be having a negative influence on society overall, as well as on the quality and quantity of sport and physical activity education programs of children and youth.

Sporting Patterns Forged by Environmental Forces

How did this happen? Phyllis Hill, in her insightful study (1965), titled

A Cultural History of Sport in Illinois, 1673-1820 concluded that:

> American cultural practices, including sport, have been forged
> by environmental forces, rather than by Anglo-Saxon tradition
> unless one claims change and innovation as distinctly Anglo-
> Saxon traits. Following this line of thought, the English
> philosophy of sport, of amateurism, of gentlemanly conduct,
> and of sport for sport's sake is inoperable in a culture where
> sport is closely tied to personal achievement and success, and
> where work ethics and sport ethics are so close as to be virtually
> indistinguishable (1965).

Hill explained further that, even though we complain about
professionalism and the related conduct of athletes, we must remember that
"halcyon amateurism" was never regarded as a value. In addition, American
institutions became less and less tied to British tradition as the settlers moved
west. Thus, she stressed that:

> The solution to American sporting problems does not lie in
> English tradition. Rather, sport in America is a cultural
> phenomenon, and its problems must be studied and resolved
> in the American tradition (1975).

Whatever the situation may be, sport has emerged as a universal social
institution that was presumably designed originally to serve humankind by
helping people to cope with an ever more complex societal life characterized
by conflict and turmoil. As Hill stated, "Its problems must be studied and
resolved in the American tradition." The question remains: How well is
society or world culture accomplishing this purpose today? As I assess the
situation today, the way the situation, this proclivity to extreme
commercialization and "technologizing" of sporting activity, along with its
violence and added elements of danger, has become one of the world's major
"blind spots". *This activity—presumably designed to serve humankind beneficially—may
be doing just the opposite! In a variety of ways, the more complex and commercial it
becomes, it is actually introducing beliefs and practices that influence participants and
spectators negatively.*

Conceptualizing the Ritual of Sport

I then sought to conceptualize this more precisely–that is, what the ritual of competitive sport means. I recalled that I had discussed the topic a while back with my good friend, now the late professor Harry M. Johnson, Ph.D., of the University of Illinois, UIUC.

Johnson stressed that sport involvement was fundamentally meant to be connected with the all-important values of human life that, in slightly different forms, are vital for all "valuable' human activities. Among these values are the following:

1. Health itself (of course),

2. The value of trying to make a contribution regardless of actual success--the value of effort itself,

3. The value of actual achievement, including excellence,

4. The value of respect for opponents,

5. The value of cooperation (i.e., one's ability to subordinate the self to the attainment of collective goals),

6. The value of fair play (i.e., respect for the rules of competition, which are universal ideally),

7. The value of orderly procedure for the settling of disputes, and

8. The value of grace in intensively competitive situations--including magnanimity in victory and the ability to accept defeat gracefully–and then try to gain victory the next time.

To continue, there can be no doubt but that the celebration of such values as these in competitive sport could have this important ritualistic quality described. We can safely say this because the goals of games and what I call *educational* sport are presumably not *intrinsically* important. However, we have increasingly decided that intrinsic importance may be given to them adventitiously—*and the absence of such "donation" has become an aberration bordering on social dislocation!*

Basically, sport is said to be "pure" when the values are practiced and celebrated for their own sake as (for example) human love and a sense of community are celebrated in quite pure form in various civic ceremonies. Thus, when sport is "pure" in this sense, it presumably renews within the performers and knowledgeable spectators specific commitments to the very values that are being displayed and appreciated in public under relatively strict rules and surveillance that guarantee the noninterference of extraneous, unevenly distributed advantages.

In other words, the "purity" of ritual in both sport and many civic ceremonies should mean that certain social values are highlighted by being removed and protected from the distracting circumstances of everyday life—handicaps and temptations as well as the inevitable involvement of immediately specific goals.

The Ritual Inherent in Sport Competition Must Not Be Corrupted

Thus, careful analysis of the developing situation should be telling us that we must most careful to see to it that the important ritual inherent in sport competition is not endangered, distorted, and corrupted—as it often is now under the following circumstances:

1. When so much emphasis is placed on winning, achievement of all the other values tends to be lost or negated.
2. When the financial rewards of advanced–level participation make sport predominantly a practical activity (rather than a ritual celebrating values for their own sake).
3. When competitive sport becomes largely entertainment for which the public

pays "top dollar" so that team owners and
competitors may be adequately compensated.

(Note: Such competition increasingly involves the
enjoyment of out-and-out brutality and
even foul play rather than being a deeply serious and
lastingly satisfying kind of activity [such as religious
ritual itself is under the finest type of situation].)

4. When too sharp a separation is made between
   the performers and the spectators (consumers).

   (Note: In other words, the game (or religious ritual!)
   played or enacted before spectators as consumers
   needs to have a relationship to the "real life" activities
   of those who look on and/or partake.

5. When there is a loss of perspective, and
   skill of a physical nature and outstanding performance
   are made exclusive or the highest of values, we forget
   that these are largely instrumental in nature.

Thus, it is what these values are presumably required for subsequently is what is truly important--that is, achievement off the playing field and enjoyment of a fine life experience through the medium of the sport contest and all that this could involve

Viewed in this way, a disinterested observer can say: "Yes, I do understand what relationship the right kind of involvement in sport and tangentially related physical activity has to the fundamental purpose of a society."

The Ritual of Sport *Is* Being Corrupted

However, just what are we permitting to happen at present? The ritual of sport is being corrupted daily. The following is a list of our "transgressions" that could be easily expanded:

1. Promoting the idea that "WINNING" is the only thing…

2. Spending infinitely more money on varsity sports for the

very few than that spent on intramural sports for the overwhelming majority

3. Offering "athletic scholarships" when there is no "financial need".

4. Permitting "trash talk" in competitive sport.

5. Permitting "showboating" by athletes after a successful play.

6. Permitting "TV sport universities" to debase education by promoting semi-professional sport played by so-called "scholar-athletes".

7. Permitting professional boxing (with the attendant brain damage!)

8. Featuring professional wrestling on television that is a disgusting sham and travesty of the fine sport of wrestling

9. Permitting "all-out" combat ("Extreme Sport") on television (and now it's offered for women too!).

10. Permitting (promoting?) the development of "high-risk" sport where "life and limb" are increasingly threatened.

11. Promoting the idea that competitive sport is good for young people, but then denying funding for intramural sport for the large majority of students in the schools.

12. Permitting professional boxing as a sport for women too!

13. Encouraging the whole idea of "martial-art" sport—when it's "self-defense" that should be stressed—not aggression!

14. Failing to take action sooner--and more strongly!— against drugs in sport. This abuse will "kill" sport in the long run… (Is this the antidote?)

15. Permitting the type of sport in which studies have shown *fair play, honesty, and sportsmanship actually decline in a university experience* (Stoll et al.).

16. Paying ridiculously high salaries to professional athletes thus creating a "false sense of values" to youth.

17. Permitting the concept of "hero" to be applied to professional athletes, an unworthy of such ascription thus unduly influencing youth as to what's important in life.

18. Overemphasizing the importance of involvement (*and winning!*) in *international* sport competition. (the "Own the podium" mentality)

19. Permitting the expansion of "violent" sports, but not also making appropriate provisions for excellent "sport injury care" for all.

20. Fostering a way of life that encourages "spectatoritis" instead of actual ongoing involvement in healthful physical activity and sport.

The Appropriate Remedies for "Errant" Sport Must Be Instituted

If these conditions are true, it means that we need to assess the evolving situation carefully and then proceed to institute the appropriate remedies. To provide us with an approach that should help to communicate with policy makers at all levels about this ever-increasing problem, consider the five–question approach to the building of effective communication skills recommended by Mark Bowden, a communications specialist (*National Post*, Canada, 2008 11 24, FP3)

Question 1: Where are we now?

The answer is that we have in so many instances permitted deviation from the basic, valuable purposes for which sport was originally created.

Osterhoudt (2006) tells us that competitive sport has become increasingly devoted to "the production, distribution, and consumption of commodities, power, wealth, fame, and privilege in predominantly medical, military, character enhancement, acculturative, political, commercial, entertainment, and recreational terms, which is to say in *instrumental* terms" (R. G. Osterhoudt in *Sport As a Form of Human Fulfillment*, Victoria, BC, CA: Trafford, 2006)).

Question 2. Why are we here?

The answer is that we are here because society has mistakenly permitted the excess of capitalistic and technological development to influence and adversely sport in the same way that other societal institutions have been influenced by these influences. Sport does indeed seem to be "the opiate of the masses"! Such development and "progress" have also joined forces with ongoing technological advancement confronting society almost irresistibly.

Question 3. Where do we want to be?

The answer is—as mentioned above—that we want to make certain that we create a situation where *"Sport involvement is related to and connected with the all-important values of human life that, in slightly different forms, are vital for all 'valuable' human activities."*

Question 4. How do we get there?

The answer is that we should be most careful to see to it, therefore, that *the important ritual inherent in sport competition* is maintained to the greatest extent possible. As we have seen, it is endangered, distorted, and corrupted by the presence of the following circumstances:

a. When so much emphasis is placed on winning, achievement of all the other values tends to be lost or negated.

b. When the financial rewards of advanced–level participation make sport predominantly a practical activity (rather than a ritual celebrating values for their own sake).

c. When competitive sport becomes largely entertainment for which the public pays "top dollar" so that team owners and competitors may be adequately compensated.

(Note: Such competition increasingly involves the enjoyment of out-and-out brutality and even foul play rather than being a deeply serious and lastingly satisfying kind of activity.)

d. When too sharp a separation is made between the performers and the spectators (consumers).

(Note: In other words, the game or context that is played or enacted before spectators or consumers needs to have a relationship to the "real life" activities of those who look on and/or partake.

e. When there is a loss of perspective, and skill of a physical nature and outstanding performance are made exclusive or the highest of values, we forget that these are largely *instrumental* in nature for the achievement of power, wealth, fame, and privilege in predominantly commercial and entertainment enterprises.

Thus, it is what these values are presumably required for subsequently is what's really important--that is, achievement off the playing field and enjoyment of a fine life experience through the medium of the sport contest and all that this could involve.

Question 5. What exactly should we do?

f. The answer is that we should encourage all professionals active in physical activity education and educational sport to place *quality* as the first priority of their professional endeavors. Their personal involvement and specialization should include a high level of competency and skill under girded by established knowledge about the highest type of aims and objectives in competitive sport that our profession should be promoting. On such a basis, it can be argued that the role of professional task sport coaches and physical activity educators is as important as any in society.

Concluding Statement

The present is no time for indecision, half-hearted commitment, imprecise knowledge, and general unwillingness to debate this position about the highest or ideal form of sport participation with the public at all levels. If we hope to bring the benefits of the *"right* kind" of sport participation to children and youth, we must sharpen our focus and improve the quality of our professional effort. Only in this way will we be able to combat the modification process that capitalistic society and accompanying technology have visited upon us in respect to people's understanding of what constitutes the finest type of competitive sport. In the 21st century, humankind deserves better than the type of sport as a social institution that "somehow" gradually materialized in the 20th century.

Chapter 4
Competitive Sport Was Transformed
in the Twentieth Century

The Original Enlightenment Ideal

Our chief criterion of progress has undergone a subtle but decisive change since the founding of the Republic. That change is at once a cause and a reflection of our current disenchantment with technology.

Recall that the late 18th century was a time of political revolution when monarchies, aristocracies, and the ecclesiastical structure were being challenged on a number of fronts. Also, the factory system was undergoing significant change at that time. Such industrial development with its greatly improved machinery "coincided with the formulation and diffusion of the modern Enlightenment idea of history as a record of progress. . . ."

Thus, this "new scientific knowledge and technological power was expected to make possible a comprehensive improvement in all of the conditions of life--social, political, moral, and intellectual as well as material" ([not *the*] Marx, p. 5).

This idea did slowly take hold and eventually "became the fulcrum of the dominant American worldview" (p. 5). By 1850, however, with the rapid growth of the United States especially, the idea of progress was already being dissociated from the Enlightenment vision of political and social liberation.

Technocratic Ideas and Enlightenment Ideas of Progress Clashed

By the turn of the century (1900), "the technocratic idea of progress [had become] a belief in the sufficiency of scientific and technological innovation as the basis for general progress." This came to mean that if scientific-based technologies were permitted to 0develop in an unconstrained manner, there would be an automatic improvement in all other aspects of life!

What had happened--because this theory became coupled with onrushing, relatively unbridled capitalism--was that the ideal envisioned by

Thomas Jefferson *had been turned upside down*. Instead of social progress being guided by such values as justice, freedom, and self-fulfillment for all, these goals of vital interest in a democracy were subjugated to a burgeoning society dominated by supposedly more important instrumental values.

The chief criterion of progress has undergone a subtle but decisive change since the founding of the Republic. That change is at once a cause and a reflection of some of the current disenchantment with technology. Recall that the late 18th century was a time of political revolution when monarchies, aristocracies, and the ecclesiastical structure were being challenged on a number of fronts.

Also, the factory system was undergoing significant change at that time. Such industrial development with its greatly improved machinery "coincided with the formulation and diffusion of the modern Enlightenment idea of history as a record of progress. . . ."

Hence, this "new scientific knowledge and technological power was expected to make possible a comprehensive improvement in all of the conditions of life--social, political, moral, and intellectual as well as material" ([not *the*] Marx, p. 5).

This idea did slowly take hold and eventually "became the fulcrum of the dominant American worldview" (p. 5). By 1850, however, with the rapid growth of the United States especially, the idea of progress was already being dissociated from the Enlightenment vision of political and social liberation.

By the turn of the century (1900), "the technocratic idea of progress [had become] a belief in the sufficiency of scientific and technological innovation as the basis for general progress." This came to mean that if scientific-based technologies were permitted to develop in an unconstrained manner, there would be an automatic improvement in all other aspects of life!

What had happened--because this theory became coupled with onrushing, relatively unbridled capitalism--was that the ideal envisioned by Thomas Jefferson *had been turned upside down*. Instead of social progress being guided by such values as justice, freedom, and self-fulfillment for all, these goals of vital interest in a democracy were subjugated to a burgeoning society dominated by supposedly more important instrumental values. This leaves humankind with a fundamental question: Which values will win out in the long run?

The Decline of Sport's "Mentality"

A concerned person can only be discouraged about what happened to competitive sport in the 20th century. This "decline" is continuing inexorably into the present one. I'm not talking about the drug issue, although that's a literally horrendous problem.

It could be that the best advice I could give to myself (!) might be to just *"shut up"* on the subject of the "developing sport realm". However, that wouldn't be me. I am sad to say that the "higher realm" of sport has *simply* not evolved as I hoped it would.

Many of you will get to see what happens down the line, but not me at age 90, I fear. At least I hope that sensible people "out there" will somehow be able to lessen the impact and keep the "commercial forces at bay" to a reasonable extent. I--and like-minded people of my generation--just couldn't seem to manage it.

As a youngster in New York City in the 1920s, I rooted for the Yankees with Lou Gehrig and Babe Ruth (more for the former because he was a wonderful person too). I played high school and college sport in New England in the 1930s, sport that was in perspective with life's other aspects.

Subsequently, in the 1940s and 1950s, I was involved in the coaching three sports (football and swimming or wrestling alternately at Yale and Western Ontario. It was still "educational" and "recreational" then too. I confess to even rooting for the Detroit Lions football team in the 1950s when I was teaching and coaching in Canada the first time.

When I moved to Michigan (Ann Arbor) in the late 1950s and early 1960s, however, I began to see that--even in that great university--the "tail was wagging the dog" too frequently! A Michigan professor in astronomy went on all away trips and was known as the "a-b-c lady": "A" for athletes, "B" for boys, and "C" for coeds unless they were outstanding students.

However, it was at Illinois (C-U) as department head in the 1960s, that I first encountered the cheating and under-the-table chicanery of a relatively small number of my own faculty members (coaches). And, sadly, I found I was powerless--as the department head--to even get the facts of the matter, much less have anything to say about it. The president's office took over when football and basketball "problems" erupted and became the "Illinois Slush-Fund Scandal" in 1966-67. So I decided to get out of administration fast after experiencing a duodenal spasm. If a department head can't even find out what his faculty members are being charged with--what the Hell!

Canadian "Retreat" Brings "Sanity"

Fortunately I was able to "retreat" to Canada in 1971 as dean of a new faculty (college) at The University of Western Ontario. There--for the second time--I found that I had real student-athletes in class. The first term back I didn't even know who were the varsity football and basketball athletes in my classes. (No coaches were calling me weekly either to check up as to whether their "hot dogs" were attending classes!) This made me feel "whole" again about the interrelationship of physical activity education and intercollegiate sport within education. (I'll leave that narrative at that point, although I recognize that Canada must now be alerted in this respect at the university level too. Stay half-awake if you are sleeping next to an elephant!)

So, what can I say to competitive sport in the United States as I gradually fade from the picture? I can only ask the question: Is highly competitive sport doing what will eventually mean anything of true worth to society? Does it have anything like "tenable theory" behind it to justify its presence in society at that level? Sadly I must ask "To what extent will it be possible to 'salvage' what has become an increasingly 'out-of-control' sport establishment?"

Middle schools, high schools, and colleges and universities need fine intramural & extramural sports and fitness programs. Do they have them? A reasonable number of colleges and universities do. Period! We should be both encouraging the establishment of such programs, as well as preparing fine sport and physical activity managers to administer them. I say: "Let overemphasized, commercialized sport--including the Olympic Movement and the new (ha!) 'extreme' sport--go the way of the Coliseum in ancient Rome."

Elementary and secondary educational institutions really need fine physical (activity) and health educators--not interscholastic sport coaches worrying about win-loss records that threaten their tenure. We are finding increasingly that–somehow–these coaches have never been prepared in professional preparation programs. However, we can't even guarantee that they would have been imbued with sound ethical perspectives there. Despite my extensive background in athletics and with coaching, I have finally come to believe the coaching of interscholastic athletics and inter-institutional athletics in higher education should be completely separate. It didn't have to be that way! But--purely and simply--we blew it. Now, by and large, it's a joke--or a tragedy…

Competitive Sport Must Blend With Fitness And Health Status of All

Today, at the start of the 21st century, we are beginning to truly understand the crisis in regard to the "fitness & health status" of the large majority of our youth. The welfare of these boys and girls must be paramount. Competitive sport for the "accelerated" should be promoted *only* after the welfare *of all of our youth* has been looked after adequately.

The professional sport management associations, established relatively recently have a unique opportunity to exert at least *some* influence on the future of sport through their efforts in sport management education in society. Looking to this end, I offer seven thoughts for your consideration and possible approval:

1. I believe we need to truly understand "where sport has been" and "where it is now"–if we ever hope to know "where sport should go."

2. I believe sport, as a social institution, should be doing more good than harm.

3. I believe sport and physical activity management can be a fine profession.

4. I believe that the sport and physical-activity experience should be educationally and recreationally sound.

5. I believe there is a need for developing sport and physical activity management *theory*. The blossoming profession should prove to the world what sport is or isn't doing to society.

6. I believe, also, that we need an ongoing scientific inventory of "ordered generalizations about (a) what we know and (b) what we "think we know" about the "physical activity experience" in competitive (being careful to separate the "a" & "b" categories!).

7. I believe finally that we "had better be about our business very soon" with *both* pure and applied research.

Finally, I can only say to those interested in sport management professionally, semi-professionally, or even on a voluntery basis: "Ladies and gentlemen--even though the "multitude out there"--and, indeed, many of us--don't appreciate it, "devastating storm clouds are looming…" Batten down the hatches!

Chapter 5
The Story of Siwash "U" in the Mid-1950s

This is a factual case about the football fortunes of a well-known football power in the United States about 55 years ago. All proper names have been changed to avoid embarrassment to anyone still alive who might have been involved in the program at that time (i.e., to protect both the innocent and the guilty). The basic material was taken almost completely from several national magazines, local newspapers, personal letters from close observers, and observations of associates. Thus, the sources cannot be revealed.)

The Bears Were Once an Ominous Sight

There was a time when the blue-and-gold uniforms of the Bears were an ominous sight in the Northern State Conference. During the days of old Sam Jackson (1908-16), when many colleges were still playing rugby, the State University of Siwash never lost a football game. After World War I, Jack Thompson, a rugged homegrown coach, built a formidable series of teams out of the big youths in their native region. Players like Lars Larson and the fabled Jordan brothers led Siwash into the Camelia Bowl after the 1923 and 1935 seasons, the golden era of Siwash University football. Like Larson, SU backs seemed to run over rather than around anyone brave enough to get in their way. They were truly the Bears of football.

It was symbolic of Siwash football that "hometowners" considered it sissy stuff when the college put turf on the home stadium after the arrival of Coach Jim Jenkins in 1930. The hides of the home players were so tough they had never been bothered by the sand-and-gravel surface that sent visiting teams away whining in pain. With the advent of grass there was a long dry spell in Bear football, punctured by only one Camelia Bowl visit--in 1937, when Rand State U. walloped them 21-0. Not until Burt Sanderson and Jon Blake, later to star as pros, brightened up the team in the early 1950s did Bear rooters have anything to root about, but their cheers were brief. The simple fact was that all the best SU football talent was coming from adjoining states, where Sanderson had been discovered, and Siwash wasn't getting its fair share any more.

Siwash Gets a New Coach

Joe Briggs stepped into this football void in 1953 with a huge local reputation. From 1930-32 he had been a Bear backfield star, winner in his senior year of the Standlee Medal as the "most inspirational player." Later as a high school coach in Suffridge, he had stepped out and won three championships. Then, as the Bear freshman coach for five years, his teams won 22 out of 23. So, when Coach George Graham went down the chute after a 7-3 win-loss season, the cry for Briggs was too loud to be denied. Bob Golden, the Gridiron Club president, Athletic Director Hanley Borden, and at least one member of the University board of trustees, would have preferred former Backfield Coach Rock Steckel (now at Jordan U.), but the alumni would not be denied. Briggs was hired.

Funding Good Football Players

Good football players, to put it mildly, are not easy to come by. A good team can cost $5,000 a month or more in scholarships and campus-job payments, and, when that isn't sufficient, special inducements such as convertibles and free trips home and vacation jobs and even jobs for the players' wives. Football players, if they are smart enough to learn a fake reverse, understand their own value and are quick to capitalize on it.

No one knows this better than Bob Golden, president of the Gridiron Club and a really remarkable booster in a city of boosters. Since his undergraduate days at Siwash, Bob Golden, a carrot-topped little dynamo who was a .300-hitting second baseman on the college team and president of the Big S club in his senior year, has been all for the Bears. Right after graduation in 1923, as assistant graduate manager, he started working for better football, and he doesn't mind admitting that he helped build the Camelia Bowl teams of 1924 and 1926. Nowadays Bob is Mr. Football around Siwash, and it was he that much of the conversation concerned last week.

So that good football players may enjoy the advantages of a Siwash U education, Bob Golden runs the Siwash Advertising Fund, which, as he tells it, is used "primarily for transportation costs, entertainment, and expenses for prospective athletes." Once Bob explained: "It's a fact of life that a kid can't be a college athlete and make it through school if he's in any need at all without outside help, and that's why there's a fund like ours at almost every other university."

Bob's fund is a big one--it has run in the past anywhere from $20,000 to $75,000--and he runs it pretty much as he pleases. Mostly the contributions come from 70 to 80 local big and little businessmen, labor leaders, medical doctors, lawyers, and others interested in civic betterment, people who contributed checks ranging up from fifty dollars. Now and then Bob sees a chance to make an extra pile for the fund, such as the exhibition pro football game last summer held in Siwash Stadium. The Advertising Fund netted $28,000 for this effort.

Everyone Seemed "Surprised" at the Game's Results

Everyone, particularly university and state officials, seems very surprised with this piece of information when it was finally published. No one pretended there was anything dishonest about it. They just seemed surprised that what had passed for an event to make great the city of Siwash--and a professional sports event at that--was helping put amateur football players through the local university. No doubt if they had been told about it in advance, they would have been perfectly happy. Hearing about it later was something of a shock.

Coach Joe Briggs, who was appointed in 1953, is a man who inspires fierce loyalty among his friends. Nonetheless, even by his own appraisal, he is not an easy man to be with. "I've been told I'm sarcastic, and I admit it," he said recently. "I bore down on the kids during the week so they'd be prepared for the pressure on Saturday. I goaded the kids and I needled them and I demanded discipline. I wanted Saturday to seem like a breeze to them. Let's not kid each other; there's not enough discipline anywhere today for modern kids. I think football is the last frontier of discipline."

Like any coach, Joe had his share--perhaps more--of bad luck in his first two years. There were injuries to key players at the worst time, and there were vital plays called back for penalties. Yet his real problem was that of most losing coaches, lack of good manpower. As a result he won only five of his first 20 games. Once, on a road trip to Stanton, Joe was visited at a practice session by Rex Louth, his old Bear coach, now retired. Louth watched for a while, then said: "Joe, you better get some ballplayers. You haven't got a guy on that field who's worth a newspaper photographer's time."

This was no news to Briggs, or to Golden or any of the other Bear boosters, of whom even faraway southern Dyckstra has its share. The most active of them in that area, a clique that revolves around Stanton, soon stole some of the cream of the Stanton area junior colleges right out from under the noses of such football powers as Stanton and Boulder. It was quite a haul, but as a Stanton booster observed about Siwash: "When they want a man, they get him. They dig."

Controversial Reg Branch is Hired

Not the least of Siwash's athletic harvest was Reg Branch, who had coached the great Sid Tanzer at Waterloo High School. Originally Branch had left Waterloo to go to Stanton along with Sid in what the cognoscenti call a "package deal." However, when Sid became unhappy and defected to Boulder, Branch was nevertheless kept on for another year despite his frequent criticisms of Head Coach Sands' methods to other assistant coaches. So, when Siwash hired Branch as an assistant for Briggs last spring, Branch was given an enthusiastic farewell by his fellow coaches at Stanton. For Siwash he presumably represented an attraction and a pipeline to top high school players in the Stanton area.

Branch did indeed help Briggs and his assistants come up with a good crop of recruits including some excellent junior college transfers. So, when the Bear varsity lined up against ineffectual little Statler University last September 17 for an easy opener, it was obvious to anyone who knew the ABC's of football in Siwash that this was the make-or-break year for Joe Briggs. As the game progressed, however, Briggs could hardly believe his eyes. The team fumbled 11 times for a new conference record and barely eked out a 14-7 victory. Not until the coaches had studied the game film, however, did they discover that the center had been snapping the ball a half-count too soon. Some quick detective work revealed that he had done so on the instructions of one Reg Branch. "I was just trying an experiment," Branch explained. "I wanted to fire Branch on the spot," responded Briggs, "but Hanley Borden, our AD, advised me to wait."

The Season's "Ups and Downs"
Create Pressure for Coach Briggs

For a while the Bears seemed to have regained their poise, rolling over Sparland 30-0 and upsetting powerful Boulder 7-0. Then followed two very mediocre weeks against Lanier and Douglas, and finally defeats by Lockland State and Stanton. By this time it was obvious something was terribly wrong. "I find out," stated Briggs, "that Marshall [quarterback Topper Marshall, a demoted first-stringer] is trying to persuade the most promising young quarterback on the squad to leave school. I bounced Marshall off the squad, but I wound up taking him back when [booster] Golden played sweet music on my heart strings by telling me that Marshall would lose his sponsor and also be evicted from his home. So, after he apologized to the squad, I took him back, but he went right on spreading dissension."

The first explosion came at the end of the season when a group of Bear players marched in to see Bob Golden to complain of Joe Briggs's coaching. They had signed a petition asking for his release. The coach, they said, was too strict; he would not let them ride home from games with their girlfriends; he yelled at them; he would not let them whistle in the dressing room or chew grass (!); and he made them sit erect on the bench. Citing a list of these and other complaints, the players stated that four promising freshmen had quite Siwash to solicit offers elsewhere.

Golden passed the list of complaints along to the athletic director, Hanley Borden, who passed the complaint along to the board of trustees. After a lengthy meeting, Briggs was rehired with the injunction to "straighten out his differences with his players." Anyone who knew Siwash football could have told you that Joe Briggs was through. He buried the hatchet and smoked a peace pipe with most of his players, but he was still out of grace with both Borden and Golden. What he could not patch up was his 5-4-1 record. (It is interesting to note that at the time of the revolt and the petition, pro-Briggs squad members suddenly found their mailbags empty of checks. "Players," said Joe, "had to look in two directions: one way for favors, the other for coaching."

Coach Briggs Is Fired!

Briggs received a late Xmas present--he was fired on January 27. The next day he started to talk to any and all who would listen. His righteous indignation was bursting out all over. "The filthiest thing in the world," he said, "is to corrupt young Americans with dough. I may never coach again, but, God willing, I'm not going to let them corrupt any more kids." Later he added: "I went along, all right--with the full knowledge of my superiors. No coach has any other choice under the unrealistic rules that prevail in the Western State Conference and others like it."

University Officials Declare Innocence

Interestingly, everyone else around the campus seemed quite stunned at the thought that football players were receiving extracurricular salaries. Said AD Hanley Borden: "To the best of my knowledge, no coach or myself has at any time willfully violated the conference rules. Neither I nor any member of my department has had any relationship with any so-called fund."

The president of Siwash, the eminent Harlow Standish, echoed the denial: "I want to say at once that these suggestions simply are not true." A re-echo came from Vice-President R.A. (Rick) Allen, a former president of the Western State Conference, who announced: "Were I to receive evidence that any player has been receiving anything like outside monthly payments, I would immediately declare him disqualified for team participation." The Board of Trustees? Said its chair, Mrs. R. Douglas Smythe, who with her husband, a financial consultant, are longtime friends of Hanley Borden: "I know nothing about it at all."

Chapter 6
The Illinois Slush-Fund Scandal of the 1960s

Preservation of what has been termed "the amateur ideal" has always been a problem in U.S. competitive sport at the intercollegiate level (Flath, 1964). The excesses of the early twentieth century, for example, have been amply described in the now famous Carnegie Foundation report *(American College Athletics)* which stressed that the prevailing amateur code had been violated continually (1929). In colleges and universities where gate receipts were important, these excesses have continued on unabated despite the well-meaning intentions of many who were concerned. There have been periodic investigations, books written, and commissions established, all resulting in hand-wringing and subsequent condemnation. However, these responses to the flagrant excesses have generally been to no avail.

Although it is true that these evils have been exposed actually in only a relatively few colleges and universities, intercollegiate athletics has resultantly been marred by an enormous quantity of highly unfavorable media attention. (Maybe this is so because people have a right to expect something more wholesome from institutions of higher education.) However, what has happened, and what has been reported, have strongly influenced the "atmosphere and mentality" of college and high school athletics generally. Moreover, somehow highly competitive sport in the United States has taken on a life of its own above (or below!) the espoused values and norms of the society.

The following is the story of what happened to a great educational institution in the realm of intercollegiate athletics in the late 1960s. It is called "The Illinois Slush-Fund Scandal of the 1960s." (1) The various topics included will be discussed in the following order: (a) Announcement of the "Irregularities"; (b) The Big Ten Investigation & Search for a New Athletic Director; (c) The University's Appeal & The Subsequent Decision; (d) The Search for New Coaches; (e) Results of NCAA Deliberations; and (f) Conclusions and Discussion.

Announcement of the "Irregularities

In November, 1966, Doug Mills, who had been Director of Intercollegiate Athletics at the University of Illinois for twenty-five years, decided to retire. After he resigned from his post, a search for his successor began. Pete Elliott, the Head Football Coach at Illinois, was mentioned prominently among the candidates for the position.

On December 17, 1966, it was reported that Big Ten Commissioner Bill Reed had issued the following statement on December 16 concerning Illinois' recruiting practices:

> Dr. David D. Henry, President of the University of Illinois, has reported to me Friday that there have been brought to his attention certain irregularities with respect to grants-in-aid assistance to athletes at the university.
>
> He believes that he is in possession of all the facts and has invited my inquiry into the matter with the offer of full cooperation on the part of the university in any investigation I may wish to undertake.
>
> I will begin the investigation in accordance with regular conference procedures and will have no further comment until it is completed (*The News-Gazette*, Dec. 17, 1966).

To those close to the scene, it quickly became apparent what had brought this unusual situation. Mel Brewer, the Assistant Athletic Director, learned that Pete Elliott was about to be named as the person to succeed Doug Mills, the retiring Athletic Director. Thinking about his many years of loyal service to Illinois, Brewer became extremely upset that he was not being recommended for the post. He decided to reveal to President Henry a number of infractions of the rules that had occurred, infractions in which Elliott, Harry Combes (Basketball Coach), and Howie Braun (Assistant Basketball Coach) had been involved. These rule violations in regard to financial aid presumably implicated a total of twelve tendered athletes in football and basketball (*The Daily Illini*, Dec. 17, 1964.)

The immediate aftermath of the announcement was predictable. The story became a "media bonanza" all over the country. In 1967 this story, and what subsequently transpired, was selected in the twin cities of Champaign-Urbana where the University is located, as the leading, local-event news story of the year (*The Urbana Courier*, Dec. 31, 1967). Mel Brewer offered his resignation from Intercollegiate Athletics shortly after the disclosure, even though he retained a twenty-five percent teaching responsibility with the Department of Physical Education for Men, an assignment that had been handled capably over the years. His resignation from Athletics was accepted as of January 31, 1967. Mr. Brewer was criticized in many quarters as a "Judas" because of the timing of his release of the information. Loren Tate, a local sports columnist, wrote:

> Mel Brewer, the man who drilled the holes in the side of the ship, is no longer welcome, however. His revelations have shocked a university president whose ears never should have been dented with this sort of thing. In his world, President Henry cannot be expected to comprehend the jungle that is Big Ten athletics (*The News-Gazette*, Dec. 21, 1966).

(It is somewhat difficult to accept such pontification on the part of Mr. Tate who was fully aware of the fact that intercollegiate athletics at Illinois was under the direct supervision of the President's Office. However, it must be appreciated that this affair became a sensation and a newspaper "soap opera" overnight with most of the members of the community eagerly awaiting the following day's installment. For example, three star basketball players had been declared ineligible at that time. Thus, with the entire community caught up in the developing true-life drama, the sports editors were literally in their glory as both narrators *and* oracles.) (2)

The Big Ten Investigation

On Friday, December 22, 1966 (only three days before Christmas Day!), the Big Ten and NCAA officials met for eleven hours in a closed session. Illinois officials, Vice-President Herbert Farber and Acting Athletic Director Les Bryan, submitted the actual documents that had been received by President Henry from Mr. Brewer. The next steps were for Bill Reed, the Big Ten Commissioner, to present the facts to the nine Athletic Directors for a ruling, and also for Arthur Bergstrom, Assistant Executive Director of the National Collegiate Athletic Association, to forward the evidence of the infractions to the appropriate committee for a ruling at the national level (*The Courier*, December 23, 1966).

It soon became evident that various people and representatives of the press were looking for scapegoats. For example, Bill Reed was being criticized for the suspension of the three basketball players in mid-season, but it turned out that Illinois officials had initiated a request for such a status themselves (*The Courier*, December 24, 1966). Further, Reed indicated that the University had indeed turned over a set of meticulous records indicating that a total of twenty-nine athletes had received emergency-need and/or travel payments. He stressed further that everything had been in the hands of a local businessman, and that donations to the fund had been solicited from friends and alumni of the University. The sums of money granted were actually very small, relatively speaking, a fact which caused the commissioner to remark that "I don't know why it was felt necessary to give excessive aid when legitimate loan funds are available on the campus" (*Ibid.*).

By the first of the new year (1967), it became apparent that this affair was going to have to grind itself out, and also that a new athletic director had to be chosen. Daily articles and opinion columns appeared in the three local newspapers, material that was embellished by comments from other sections of the state, region, and nation. The system was blamed; the alumni were blamed; local businessmen were blamed; the administrators were blamed; the coaches were blamed; and the athletes were blamed. A persistent theme that emerged was "others are doing it; why can't we?" An editorial in *The Daily Illini* complained that "The United States is the only nation in the world which tries to uphold this idealistic attitude toward amateur athletics. If our rules governing amateurs were in line with those of other nations, we would walk away with almost every gold medal at the Olympics . . . (January 5, 1967).

In an interesting issue of *The Daily Illini*, dated Jan. 14, 1967, the headline stated "Big Questions Still Unanswered," and then Dan Balz, the sports editor, proceeded to delineate what he called "new facts and statements." For example, he stated that Mel Brewer had had no direct contact with President Henry, and that he had simply reported the fact to Les Bryan, the acting athletic director, on December 7. Further, he stated that there were three, not two, illegal funds as had been reported earlier. The "books" on these funds had presumably been kept by Bill Burrows, an employee of Bailey and Himes, a local sporting goods company, and also presumably "on the request of Doug Mills, former athletic director." Still further, Balz reported that "many of the payments made to the athletes would have been approved, had they gone through legitimate channels." Finally, Balz stated that it was known that "the athletes received no hearing before they were suspended" (*The Daily Illini*, Jan. 14, 1967, p. 1).

In the meantime, a number of different names were being mentioned as possibilities for the vacant post of athletic director. Gene Vance, 43-year old alumni director of the University, was named as the fourth athletic director in the university's history. Vance was indeed a member of the "Illinois family," having played guard on two championship basketball teams in 1942 and 1943 with Doug Mills as his head coach. While waiting until April 1, the date when he was scheduled to assume the position, he planned to "spend time with Dr. Bryan to get background on the situation and talk to the coaches and their staffs" (*The News-Gazette*, January 17, 1967).

For the next five to six weeks, the local and regional newspapers were full of reports, statements, counter-statements, rumors, letters to the editor, and similar items. In his annual "State of the University Report", President Henry wrote "I am deeply disappointed that representatives of the Athletic Association have been responsible for infractions of the regulations of the Intercollegiate (Big Ten) Conference . . . No university can tolerate a double standard in keeping its agreements" (*The Urbana Courier*, Jan. 21, 1967). Exactly one month later (February 22, 1967), President Henry learned that the Big Ten Athletic Directors agreed with him strongly. The directors voted to force Illinois to dismiss the three coaches involved (Elliott, Combes, and Braun).

President Henry, after discussing the matter with the University's legal counsel, James J. Costello, immediately announced his intention to appeal what he considered to be a "too harsh" penalty. Such an appeal had to be made to the final arbiters, the faculty representatives of the Big Ten. It was this group that also had the responsibility of deciding what would happen to the twelve athletes who had been declared ineligible by the University itself when the violations had been disclosed *(The Urbana Courier*, February 23, 1967).

The University's Appeal; The Subsequent Decision

Even though there was no reason to think that any ruling would be a light one, so to speak, and even though the "show cause" rule (as it was called) indicated that a university's membership in the conference could be terminated or suspended for infractions, most university officials and others involved in some way with Illinois felt the ruling was too harsh, was unfair, and represented a "crushing blow" to the university's athletic future (*The*

News-Gazette, Feb. 23, 1967). However, an editorial in *The Daily Illini* ended with the following words: "It often is harder to acknowledge that a good friend has done something wrong. But when the evidence is there, there is little room for discussion. We agree with the Big Ten" (February 24, 1967). Another column written by Bob Strohm was entitled "Misplaced Loyalty." It refers to "Captain Henry." and stated the following: "As for the childish rationalizations conjured up by almost everyone under the spell of 'spunky' Dr. Henry (that) 'Everyone else is doing it; why should we get punished?' That brand of thought is most often heard by grade school teachers" *(Ibid.)*.

Based on the ensuing publicity--although others expressing similar opinions most often declined to be named (!)--it was obvious that *The Daily Illini* and a few others were in the minority. Two different petitions urging that the coaches be retained were circulated by some alumni and some football players. The president of the Illinois High School Coaches' Association moved to get the state's coaches behind the University's appeal (*The News Gazette*, February 25, 1967). All eighty-two members of the football squad signed a petition. The Board of Directors of the Athletic Association met to affirm its support of the coaches. Hal McCoy in *The Detroit Free Press* stated "It's not Illinois on trial. It's the Big Ten . . ." (February 25, 1967). In the Illinois State Legislature, the House debated a resolution asking for leniency, but finally decided that the legislature shouldn't get involved at that point *(The News-Gazette*, March 2, 1967). Even the Honorable Otto Kerner, Governor of Illinois, took up the cause for Illinois. "I know Pete Elliott particularly. There's no finer, cleaner man. If my son were at the University and were working under Pete Elliott, I would be delighted. He's the type of man I'd like my son to associate with" (*The Urbana Courier*, February 27, 1967). (Interestingly, but sadly, the Governor himself went to jail as the result of a race track scandal and pay-off a bit later.)

All of the pleas were in vain, however, because on March 3, 1967, the faculty representatives of the Big Ten Conference sent a telegram to President Henry stating that the Commissioner be notified by March 17 whether the three coaches would be retained. "If the answer is 'no' the case is closed. If the answer to the question is 'yes' as to any of these coaches, will you discuss with the commissioner dates convenient for a hearing at which the university is invited to show cause why its membership in the conference should not be suspended or terminated?" (*The Urbana Courier*, March 4, 1967. On the next day, two basketball players, Rich Jones and Ron Dunlop were declared permanently ineligible, as was football halfback, Cyril Pinder, and four other unnamed athletes (*The News-Gazette*, March 5, 1967).

It wasn't all over yet. On Monday, March 7, Henry issued a statement that he intended to carry the matter through with a final appeal on the March 17 deadline that he had been given. Governor Kerner expressed his support for Illinois again, and the entire Board of Trustees backed the President's stance as well. Then, if matters weren't bad enough, Irv Kupcinet, a Chicago columnist, reported that Doug Mills, the retired athletic director, told him that Henry "knew as much about the fund as I did" (*The Sun-Times*, March 12, 1967). Mills denied this immediately saying that Kupcinet had misinterpreted him. "Nothing could be farther from the truth. There is no more honest man than Dr.Henry (*The News-Gazette*, March 13, 1967). No matter who was right, who was wrong, who was misinterpreted, and who wasn't, the absolutely final appeal was denied by the Big Ten Conference. "If after March 21 (Tuesday), coaches Elliott, Combes, and Braun, or any one of them, be retained . . . the membership of the University of Illinois . . . shall be suspended as of that date . . . (*The News-Gazette*, March 19, 1967).

Thus, what had seemed almost inevitable occurred on March 21--the three coaches filed their resignations. Their statement expressed deep appreciation for the support that they had received from President Henry and "alumni, students, faculty, and friends" of the University, but no mention was made of the violations of the rules by any of them. The coaches hoped that their resignations would result in the "amelioration of the penalties imposed on the students . . ." (*The Urbana Courier*, March 20, 1967).

The Search for New Coaches

Although some may disagree, it could be argued that what happened after this is almost completely anticlimactic in nature. Tate stated that "the coaches took the honorable route" (*The News-Gazette*, March 20, 1967), whereas on the same day, Bertine made the same assessment and wrote a second column in which he discussed "the many questions left in the wake of the coaches' resignations" (*The Urbana Courier*, March 20, 1967). It was explained that the search for new coaches had already begun, and that "this job will become the first major responsibility of Gene Vance when he assumes the athletic directorship on April l" (*The News-Gazette*, March 20, 1967). Even the histories of the three coaches were traced at length in *The*

Urbana Courier (March 20, 1967). (Since all of these were separate articles, one wonders what space was left for any other news in the newspapers on this day.)

On the next day (March 21, 1967), *The Daily Illini* told about a highly condemnatory editorial in *The Chicago Tribune* criticizing the Big Ten itself for its hypocritical action "when all the men have academic standing in the school of physical education." (One interesting sidelight at that time was that a mammoth testimonial dinner was held in Champaign-Urbana for the three coaches and their wives in which an unnamed co-chairman stated that "Our goal is to raise $10,000 cash for each of the three coaches. We can't do enough for these men," *The Chicago Tribune*, March 23, 1967. Each of the wives received a star-sapphire wristwatch at this dinner, and there was also discussion of starting a fund to have statues of the three coaches erected in a prominent location!)

Shortly thereafter, the new head coaches for football and basketball were announced. They were James Valek, who was immediately released by South Carolina, and Harve Schmidt, who was also immediately released from the University of New Mexico. Loren Tate, in *The News-Gazette* stated boldly "Two former University of Illinois athletics greats have been designated to lead the Fighting Illini out of the 'slush fund' quagmire" (March 29, 1967). Illinois had decided to stay within its own "athletic family."

Results of NCAA Deliberations

It was not until May 7, 1967 that the National Collegiate Athletic Association announced its decision about possible penalties to be imposed upon the University of Illinois. As might have been expected, the NCAA decided that Illinois would be barred from Rose Bowl consideration for two years, and further that there would be no post-season competition in basketball. The biggest concern in athletic circles in the Champaign-Urbana area seemed to be that this might be disappointing to the athletes and thereby cut down on their incentive to win. Further, it was felt that recruiting for the next few years would be hampered as well (*The Urbana Courier*, May 8, 1967). On top of this, just eleven days later, the faculty representatives of the Big Ten Conference denied a petition asking for modification of the ineligibility penalties against certain of the athletes involved (*The News-Gazette*, May 19, 1967). Then, on April 24, a committee of the Illinois State

Legislature brought forward a 180-page draft report recommending that Big Ten and NCAA investigations should be independent of one another "as this is not a country designed as were the occupied countries of the collaborationist Hitler regime" (*The News-Gazette*, May 24, 1967). (It will be left to the reader's imagination to decipher that enigmatic statement.)

Conclusions and Discussion

A narrative such as this must be concluded at some point, although it should be stated again that many ramifications of this unpleasant situation simply could not be included in what must be considered to be a preliminary analysis. Nevertheless, a study of this type should necessarily arrive at some conclusions and offer further discussion. Although further study may either substantiate or correct what will now be said, the following thoughts seem to be reasonable ones at this point:

Conclusions:

1. Breaking the rules has a "long history" in U.S. intercollegiate athletics.

2. The social forces at work (e.g., the society's values and norms) are evidently not sufficiently strong to permanently rectify the illegal and dishonorable situation that prevails in the gate-receipt sports throughout the land (see discussion below).

3. Inasmuch as the amateur/professional controversy has consistently been marred by illogicality and inconsistency, the possibility and practicality of "legal semi–professionalism" should be considered as one way out of this ongoing highly serious societal problem.

4. Humans under pressure reveal frailties in all types of situations, including those that arise in intercollegiate athletics. The people involved at Illinois are seemingly no better and no worse than others involved in such practices in the past and at present. Although the three coaches *and* others "sinned, these transgressions were venial, not mortal, in nature."

5. It will undoubtedly take unusual, outstanding individual and collective leadership to resolve the longstanding, shameful situation in intercollegiate athletics that makes a mockery of *espoused* national ideals, not to mention what it does to the "soul" of those colleges and universities that are involved.

Discussion:

Finally, it can be stated that we simply do not seem to learn from past mistakes. For example, in 1981 Illinois was again placed on a three years' probation by unanimous vote of the Big Ten Conference's faculty representatives. Further, even as this paper was being prepared, fresh, new penalties are to be imposed on Illinois in 1984-85. One can only speculate as to whether such travesties exhibited in the name of higher education will ever end.

It is important to say that this historical summary and analysis relates the trials and tribulations *of one university only* in the sphere of intercollegiate athletics. Obviously, there have been and are many others caught in the throes of so-called *amateur* sport that--when you get right down to it--is really *semi-professional.* However, it must be said also that what has been stated here *cannot* be regarded as representative of what goes on in competitive sport in the large majority of colleges and universities in North America (i.e., the outright cheating and defiance). For them, intercollegiate sport is still a socially useful servant in the education of both young men and (now) young women. For their sake--*for our culture's sake!*--this type of smear or blot on sport's escutcheon cannot be tolerated indefinitely. In the United States especially, "present-day slaves doing combat in the arena deserve a far better fate in the land of the free and home of the brave." To conclude, "if men could learn from history, what lessons it might teach us" (Coleridge).

Reference Notes

1. Any historical study has limitations. In this study it must be explained that the investigator was the head of the Department of Physical Education for Men (and Graduate Chairman) at the University of Illinois, Champaign-Urbana, from 1964-1968. (He decided to "get out" of administration at that point.)There are points within this narrative where some personal reference might have been made to a letter written to a dean, a comment made in response to a reporter's question, what would have been said at a committee

meeting held by the Illinois State Legislature if such a statement had been permitted, what was told to him "off the record," etc., but these were insignificant and tangential only in the drama that was unfolding. Every effort has been made to keep personal bias from this paper. Further, appreciation should be expressed to Dr. Melvin Adelman, The Ohio State University, for his assistance in the collating of data during the time when these incidents were taking place. However, he is not responsible for any opinions, errors, or omissions in this narrative.

2. It is interesting to note here that people on campus in administrative posts were *in no way* kept informed on the developments taking place. This is the main reason why this investigator kept such a careful record *through the three newspapers* of what was transpiring. It is also interesting to conjecture why the reporters were kept so well informed, while campus administrators with a legitimate claim to knowledge were told absolutely nothing. Even though the three coaches, and sixteen others, were on his departmental budget anywhere from ten to seventy-five percent (and a number of these men held university tenure), this investigator had no way of knowing what was occurring and to what extent the department's reputation might become tarnished in the process. Despite a series of letters and memoranda sent to others who might enlighten departmental personnel, no satisfactory responses were received. (A copy of a detailed letter sent on February 27, 1967 asking for tangible information is available from the investigator upon request.)

References

Carnegie Foundation for the Advancement of Teaching, *The. American college athletics*. (H. J. Savage *et al.*, eds.). New York: The Foundation, Bulletin #23, 1929.

Chicago Tribune, The, March 23, 1967.

Courier, The (Urbana), Dec. 23, 1966, Dec. 24, 1966, Jan. 21, 1967, Feb. 27, 1967, March 4, 1967, March 20, 1967, May 8, 1967, Dec. 31, 1967.

Daily Illini, The. Dec. 17, 1966, Jan. 5, 1967, Jan. 14, 1967, Feb. 24, 1967, March 21, 1967.

Detroit Free Press, The, Feb. 25, 1967.

Flath, A. W. *A history of the relations between the National Collegiate Athletic Association and the Amateur Athletic Union of the United States (1905-1963)*. Champaign, IL: Stipes

Publishing Co., 1964.

News-Gazette, The, Dec. 17, 1966, Dec. 21, 1966, Jan. 10, 1967, Jan. 17, 1967, Feb. 23, 1967, Feb. 25, 1967, March 2, 1967, March 5, 1967, March 13, 1967, March 19, 1967, March 20, 1967, March 22, 1967, March 29, 1967, May 24, 1967.

Chapter 7
Rebellion at the Canadian Interuniversity Sport Level: Implications for Financial Aid to All Students

Any intelligent observer cannot help wonder about competitive sport's place in society today. Considering the obvious excesses of commercialized sport, we could argue that increasingly they seem to be emulating the level of the Circus Maximus era of ancient Rome. (Those athletes back then often died, however, instead of becoming millionaires...)

The term "sport" has become ubiquitous. Highly commercialized sport is indeed "light years" away from the initial sporting experience of a young girl or boy facing juvenile competition for the first time.

Have you ever wondered, for example, why fans in the Canadian Football League's Toronto, Calgary, or Vancouver teams, get all excited about watching talented, but basically second-level Americans athletes represent their cities' honor in gridiron battle? What motivates these fans? We know what motivates the athletes.

The Role of Sport & Physical Recreation In Canadian University Life

Now direct your attention to the role of competitive sport and physical recreation in Canadian university life. All students should have a fine *intramural* sport and physical recreation program available to them. In addition, in North America, as opposed to the rest of the world, competitive, *extramural* sport programs for men, and then for women as well, developed within the universities themselves during the 20th century.

This development has been good, but disturbing problems have risen along the way. Canada's geography and the ever-present concern about "sleeping with an elephant" (in this case the National Collegiate Athletic Association of the USA) have become problems of immediate concern.

Why Are Some Universities Considering Secession from Canadian Interuniversity Sport?

Thus, the question is being asked today: "Why are the Thunderbirds of the University of British Columbia and the Clan of Simon Fraser University considering a move to secede from Canadian Interuniversity Sport. Both universities are considering affiliation with Division II of the National Collegiate Athletics Association in the United States?"

Is it just a question of "easier access" to opponents by heading south instead of traveling far across the Canadian terrain? Is it that NCAA Division II status allows student-athletes to receive aid that includes the costs of tuition and fees, room and board, books and supplies, and other expenses related to attendance at the University?

Why should UBC and SFU not move to Division I status in the States? Who wants to be a second-class citizen? The answer to that is simple. Division I involvement in the NCAA amounts to students becoming professional athletes. Division IA is only a short step behind. ?

The approach of Canadian University Sport (CIS) is dull, you see. It does not permit purely athletic scholarships. However, each university seems to have figured out its own unique way of assisting "scholar-athletes" to "some extent or another" This despite the CIS stipulation that financial aid is limited for student-athletes to tuition and fees only.

Consider this information from the discussion guide recently made available to members of the UBC university community in Vancouver:

> UBC athletics and recreation is dedicated to attracting the best student-athletes from around the world and considers athletic scholarships as an integral part of this plan.

> UBC's Millennium Breakfast is the largest single-day athletic scholarship fundraiser in Canada and has raised in excess of $5 million since 2000. Funds raised through this event go directly into UBC's Athletic Scholarship Endowment, which ensures that athletes have opportunities to realize their athletic and academic goals in Canada for decades to come.

73

UBC's Athletic Scholarship Endowment is approximately $9 million. While the Athletic Scholarship Endowment is used to fund athletic
scholarships, the UBC varsity teams, as well as the Department as a whole, are funded through student fees (40%) and business operations (60%), which is revenue generated through facility rental, sport camps, sponsorship and fundraising.

Donors to the Athletic Scholarship Endowment are connected to UBC Athletics and Recreation through sport — 90% of donors are former university, national or international athletes and the remaining 10% are connected in some way to a current or former varsity athlete.

UBC is in contact with more than 9,000 athletic alumni who are essential to UBC Athletics and Recreation's campaign to raise $75 million for the Athletic Scholarship Endowment over the next 10 years, which will further enhance UBC's athletic program.

This is impressive, you might say at first glance. However, if you compare the finances to that of Division I universities in the U.S.A., it is "chicken-feed". The annual budget for athletics at The Ohio State University is about 121 million dollars. The head football coach at the University of Tennessee earns $2,200,000 annually. That is big business!

The athletics department at OSU typically contributes a million dollars to the University's operating budget after paying its own expenses. The university president there "minds his p's and q's" before issuing a directive to the athletics department. It could have *him* fired if he tried to upset their applecart in any way.

It becomes obvious that we are talking about different kinds of sport in different universities. It appears that individual involvement in sport assumes different characteristics as it runs the gamut of a spectrum–from frivolity to play to competition to work!

What Is This Ritual Involving Competitive Sport?

Trying to figure this all out more precisely–that is, what the ritual of competitive sport means–I got together a while back with my good friend, now the late professor Harry M. Johnson, Ph.D., of the University of Illinois. After a series of "fireside chats," we concluded that sport involvement should be connected with the all-important values of human life that, in slightly different forms, are vital for all "valuable' human activities.

Among these values are the following:

1. Health itself (of course),

2. The value of trying to make a contribution regardless of actual success--the value of effort itself,

3. The value of actual achievement, including excellence,

4. The value of respect for opponents,

5. The value of cooperation (i.e., one's ability to subordinate the self to the attainment of collective goals),

6. The value of fair play (i.e., respect for the rules of competition, which are universalistic ideally),

7. The value of orderly procedure for the settling of disputes, and

8. The value of grace in intensively competitive situations--including magnanimity in victory and the ability to accept defeat gracefully–and then try to gain victory the next time.2

To continue, there can be no doubt but that the celebration of such values as these (immediately above) in competitive sport has this important ritualistic quality described. We can safely say this because the goals of games and what is called *educational* sport are presumably not *intrinsically* important. However, we decided that intrinsic importance may be given to them adventitiously–and the absence of such "donation" has become an aberration bordering on social dislocation.

Basically, sport is said to be "pure" when the values are practiced and celebrated for their own sake as (for example) human love and a sense of community are celebrated in quite pure form in various civic ceremonies. Thus, when sport is "pure" in this sense, it presumably renews within the performers and knowledgeable spectators specific commitments to the very values that are being displayed and appreciated in public under relatively strict rules and surveillance that serves to guarantee the noninterference of extraneous, unevenly distributed advantages.

In other words, the "purity" of ritual in both civic ceremonies and sport means that certain social values are highlighted by being removed and protected from the distracting circumstances of everyday life--handicaps and temptations as well as the inevitable involvement of immediately specific goals.

The Ritual Inherent in Sport Competition Must Not Be Corrupted

So, it can be argued successfully through careful analysis that we must be most careful to see to it that the important ritual inherent in sport competition is not endangered, distorted, and corrupted under the following circumstances:

> 1. When so much emphasis is placed on winning, achievement of all the other values tends to be lost or negated.

> 2. When the financial rewards of advanced–level participation make sport predominantly a practical activity (rather than a ritual celebrating values for their own sake).

3. When competitive sport becomes largely
entertainment for which the public
pays "top dollar" so that team owners and
competitors may be adequately compensated.

(Note: Such competition increasingly involves the
enjoyment of out-and-out brutality and
even foul play rather than being a deeply serious and
lastingly satisfying kind of activity [such as religious ritual
itself is under the finest type of situation].)

4. When too sharp a separation is made between the
performers and the spectators (consumers).

(Note: In other words, the game (or religious ritual!)
played or enacted before spectators or consumers needs
to have a relationship to the "real life" activities of those
who look on and/or partake.

5. When there is a loss of perspective, and
skill of a physical nature and outstanding performance
are made exclusive or the highest of values, we forget that
these are largely instrumental in nature.

*Thus, it is what these values are presumably required for
subsequently is what's really important--that is, achievement off the
playing field and enjoyment of a fine life
experience through the medium of the sport contest and all that this
could involve.*

Viewed in this way, a disinterested observer can say: "Yes, I do see
what relationship this has to the fundamental purpose of a university
wherever it is located in Canada?" I can understand how such experience is
part of what a university education all about.

Why Are Athletes Being Singled Out for Special Attention?

However, the question remains as to why athletes only are being singled out for "special attention" financially, when students with other, but equally important talents, are not rewarded in the same fashion.

Young people coming to universities, in addition to their knowledge, competencies, and skills acquired in their prior educational experiences, bring with them quality experiences in other educationally related aspects of life that have been deemed worthwhile traditionally.

These "quality experiences" in educationally related areas include: (1) aesthetic and creative activities, (2) communication activities, (3) social activities, (4) ancillary educational activities, AND (5) sport activities. They are all important. Students with these backgrounds help to create a vital, vibrant university community.

These young men and women come from families with varying financial backgrounds. After gaining admission, and as along as they remain bona fide students, they deserve an opportunity to experience a university education free from ever-present financial worries. In addition, after graduation they should not have to contend with staggering future debt incurred during this period when they are acquiring the background for future employment.

Universities Should Make an Even Greater Ongoing Commitment to Student Financial Aid

Universities should be commended, of course, for their ongoing commitment to help all academically qualified citizens and permanent residents to achieve their educational goals as free from financial concerns as possible. With Canada's approach to multiculturalism, the need to build on this commitment looms even larger.

At Western, for example, the four methods of financial assistance available include (1) OSAP and other government assistance programs, (2) Bursaries (Admissions and In-Course), (3) Government Assistance Program, and (4) Work Study. The following data is taken from the University's website:

OSAP provides financial assistance for educationalcosts and basic living expenses to students in postsecondary education. The amount of OSAP assistance awarded is determined by comparing educational costs (such as tuition fees, books, and basic living expenses) and personal resources (such as parental income, summer and study period income, scholarships and awards, and assets). OSAP applications are available in the spring for the upcoming September study period.

Admission Bursaries: These bursaries are non-repayable, taxable grants awarded on the basis of financial need for entering first-year students. Admission Bursaries generally range in value from $250 to $3,000. To be eligible for bursary assistance, you must be a Canadian citizen or a permanent resident, and you must demonstrate financial need. Information on how to apply for an Admission Bursary is provided when Western acknowledges your admission application with a package in the mail).

In-Course Bursaries: Bursary assistance is also available to students after first-year if they continue to have financial need. To be eligible, you must be a Canadian citizen or a permanent resident, and must complete a financial need application that is available each year in August.

Government Assistance Program Student Financial Services also administers other government assistance programs, such as the Part-Time Canada Student Loan Program, Canada Study Grant for High-Need Part-Time Students Program, and the Bursary for Students with Disabilities Program.

Work Study: Over 2,000 on-campus employment opportunities are available each year through Work Study to allow upper-year students to work in flexible environments, gain experience, and contribute financially to their education-related expenses. Students have achieved success working in laboratories, designing Web pages, writing journals, and assisting in the administration of the university. To qualify for the Work Study program, you must be a Canadian citizen or a permanent resident enrolled in at least a 60 per cent course load, and you must have financial need. Online applications are available each year in August.

The "Playing Field" Should Be Level For All Canadians in Higher Education

Candidates for admission should be evaluated without the need for financial help arising. Financial aid should be based solely on demonstrated need. The full, *demonstrated* financial need of every qualified student admitted should be met. *There should be no need for merit scholarships and athletic scholarships.*

If such a plan were implemented, monetary grants to low-income and middle-income families would increase significantly. In addition, students would find that the amount they must contribute from their own earnings would decrease. In addition to money earned from summer employment, additional funds can be earned *from no more than 10 hours of on- or off-campus employment.* There should be no need to work longer or to take out monetary loans.

Concluding Statement

The writer submits that this proposal is not radical. It is forward looking and should be implemented at the first possible moment. Qualified young people of today should not be burdened with financial problems during the vital university period. They should not have to be looking for dubious athletic scholarships in the States *or in Canada.*

Provincial governments, universities, foundations, alumni, and business should commit at this time to create an ideal situation for *all* qualified people to obtain full benefit from the university experience.

Chapter 8
"Socio-Instrumental" Values *and* "Moral" Values Converged to "Do 'Tiger' In"!

The Occurrence

Tiger Woods, named the outstanding golf professional of the 2000-2009 decade and undoubtedly a "golden boy" in the sporting world, has been leading a double life. Presumably happily married to a beautiful Swedish wife with two lovely children, and on the way to becoming fabulously wealthy, Woods had an automobile accident outside of his home in the early hours of a morning. This mishap subsequently brought to light a tale of extraordinary, "extracurricular" sexual activity with many mistresses far and wide.

This scandal immediately became one of the top media stories of the year 2009. The public was surprised and also startled. In fairly short order, the "miscreant" felt constrained to offer a public apology and to take an indefinite leave from his work as professional gold player. The implications resulting from this move away from the "world of golf" were potentially devastating to both the future of Woods himself and to the development of the sport of golf.

Why Was This Story So Newsworthy?

Watching this scandal mature over several months, I asked myself: "Why was this such a 'big deal'?" Is this development so unusual in the history of the world? Haven't various media personalities, including sport figures, experienced problems of this type before? Why is this particular incident worthy of all this attention? (*Note:* The ethical aspect of his relationship with Dr. Galea in Toronto who administered PEDs in Toronto to speed up Tiger's recovery from knee surgery is not considered here.) The answer is that this incident is not *unique*, but it is *unusual*. Yet, one wonders why has so much public attention been given to this particular situation? I believe the answer can be found in the fact that, in the past one hundred years, the role of sport in society has changed so radically. Competitive sport has gradually, but steadily, become a *social institution* that surged enormously in importance. Hence, it has become an extremely powerful social force that must be reckoned with from here into the indeterminate future.

Because of this upsurge in sport's development, I have personally been attempting to analyze it from a socio-cultural perspective. It appears to be a question of the "use of" and the "abuse of" of sport. The underlying theoretical argument that can be made is as follows: Strong institutions (i.e., "forces" or "influences") govern society. Among those social institutions are:

(1) society's values (including created norms based on these
    values),
(2) the type of political state in vogue,
(3) the prevailing economic system,
(4) the religious beliefs present, etc.

To these longstanding institutions, I have over the years added such other influences as education, the communication media, science and technological advancement, concern for peace, *and now sport itself*. Of all of these, the *values* a society holds, and the accompanying norms developed on the basis of these values, form the strongest institution of all!

Hard Questions About Present Social Institutions

Social institutions are created and nurtured within a society ostensibly to further the positive development of the people living within that culture. Take democracy, for example, as a type of political institution that is currently being promoted vigorously by the United States throughout the entire world. (Of course, such worldwide change will take time!) Within this form of social development, democracy has also developed a strong relationship with economics—especially with the institution of capitalism. Economics, of course, is another vital social institution upon which a society depends fundamentally.

As world civilization developed, a great many of the world's countries have enacted with almost messianic zeal the promotion of such social institutions as democracy, capitalism, and--now--an increasing involvement with the promotion of competitive sport. The "theory" behind such promotion is that the addition of highly competitive sport to this mix will bring about more "good" than "bad" for the people and the countries involved. However, this social experiment has raised a number of disturbing questions that society must consider.

Underlying the rampant promotion of commercialized sport, of course, is this possibly questionable alliance of democracy and rampant capitalism. Think of the example being set in North America, for example. Is there reasonable hope that this present brand of "democratic capitalism" that uses up the world's environmental resources inordinately will somehow improve the world situation in the long run? Can we truly claim with any degree of certainty that this "mix" of democracy and capitalism (with its subsequent inclusion of big-time sport) is producing more "good" than "bad"? (Admittedly, we do need to delineate between "what's 'good'" and "what's 'bad'" more carefully). There is no escaping the fact that the gap economically between the rich and the poor is steadily increasing. This means that "the American dream for all"–what was known as "the Enlightenment Ideal"–is beginning to look like a desert mirage for the "good, old USA".

What Happened to the "Enlightenment Ideal"?

Recall that the late 18th century was a time of political revolution when monarchies, aristocracies, and the ecclesiastical structure were being challenged on a number of fronts. In addition, the factory system was undergoing significant change at that time. Such industrial development with its greatly improved machinery "coincided with the formulation and diffusion of the modern Enlightenment idea of history as a record of progress. . . ." Hence, this "new scientific knowledge and technological power was expected to make possible a comprehensive improvement in all of the conditions of life--social, political, moral, and intellectual as well as material" ([Leo] Marx).

This idea did slowly take hold and eventually "became the fulcrum of the dominant American worldview" (p. 5). By 1850, however, with the rapid growth of the United States especially, *the idea of progress was already being dissociated from the Enlightenment vision of political and social liberation.* Then, by the turn of the century (1900), "the technocratic idea of progress [had become] a belief in the sufficiency of scientific and technological innovation as the basis for general progress." This came to mean that if scientific-based technologies were permitted to develop in an unconstrained manner, there would be an automatic improvement in all other aspects of life!

What had happened--because this theory became coupled with onrushing, unbridled capitalism--was that the ideal envisioned by Thomas Jefferson *had been turned upside down*! Instead of social progress being guided by *such values as justice, freedom, and self-fulfillment for all*, these goals of vital interest in a democracy were subjugated to a burgeoning society dominated by supposedly more important *instrumental* values.

As it developed, America's chief criterion of progress has undergone a subtle but decisive change since the founding of the Republic. That change is at once a cause and a reflection of much of the current disenchantment by many with advancement in technology. Hence, the fundamental question today could well be: "Which values will win out in the long run?" Will the historical "Enlightenment Ideal" remain as an unfulfilled dream forever?

Challenging the Role of Sport in Society

Now, returning to "the Tiger Woods Saga", we find Tiger as a prominent figure in sport, a social institution whose influence has increased phenomenally. This development has become so vast that we may now ask whether it is accomplishing what it is presumably supposed to do. Is highly competitive sport as a social phenomenon doing more good than harm in society? The world seems to have accepted as fact that it is! Yet the world community does not really know whether this contention is true or not. Sport's expansion is permitted and encouraged almost without question in all quarters. "Sport is good for people, and more involvement with sport of almost any type--extreme sport, professional wrestling, missed martial arts, 'world cups'—even watching it regularly (!)--is better" seems to be the conventional wisdom. Witness, in addition, the billions of dollars that are being removed neatly out of tax revenues for the several Olympic enterprises perennially.

As I analyzed the "Tiger Woods Saga," I found it impossible to avoid a critique of commercialized sport as well. I believe that the development is now such that society should be striving to keep sport's drawbacks and/or excesses in check to the greatest possible extent. In recent decades we have witnessed the rise of sport throughout the land to the status of a fundamentalist religion. For example, we find sport being called upon to serve as a "redeemer of wayward youth," but--as it is occurring elsewhere—I believe it is also becoming a destroyer of certain fundamental values of individual and social life.

Wilcox, for example, in his empirical analysis, challenged "the widely held notion that sport can fulfill an important role in the development of national character." He stated: "the assumption that sport is conducive to the development of positive human values, or the 'building of character,' should be viewed more as a belief rather than as a fact." He concluded that sport did "provide some evidence to support a relationship between participation in sport and the ranking of human values" (1991, pp. 3, 17, 18, respectively).

Assuming Wilcox's view has reasonable validity, those involved in any way in the institution of sport--if they all together may be considered a collectivity--should contribute a quantity of redeeming social value to our North American culture, not to mention the overall world culture (i.e., a quantity of good leading to improved societal well-being). On the basis of this argument, the following two questions can be postulated for response by concerned agencies and individuals (e.g., federal governments, state and provincial officials, philosophers in the discipline and related professions):

(1) Can, does, or should a great (i.e., leading) nation produce great sport?

(2) With the world being threatened environmentally in a variety of ways, should we now be considering the "ecology" of sport as we are doing with other human activity? Both the beneficial and disadvantageous aspects of a particular sporting activity should be studied through the endeavors of scholars in various disciplines as well?

(3) If it is indeed the case that the guardian of the "functional satisfaction" resulting from sport is (a) the sports person, (b) the spectator, (c) the businessperson who gains monetarily, (d) the sport manager, and, in some instances, (e) educational administrators and their respective governing boards, then who in society should be in a position to be the most knowledgeable about the immediate objectives and long range aims of sport and related physical activity?

Answering these questions is a complex matter. First, as stated above, sport and related physical activity have become an extremely powerful social force in society. Secondly, if we grant that sport now has significant power in almost all of the world's developed cultures--a power indeed that appears to be growing--we should also recognize that any such social force affecting society is dangerous if perverted (e.g., through an excess of nationalism or commercialism). With this in mind, I am stating further that sport has somehow achieved such status as a powerful societal institution without an adequately defined underlying theory. Somehow, most countries seem to be proceeding generally on a typically unstated assumption that "sport is a good thing for society to encourage, and *more* sport is even better!" And yet, as explained above, the term "sport" exhibits radical ambiguity based on both everyday usage and dictionary definition. This obviously adds even more to the present problem and accompanying confusion.

This "radical ambiguity" about the role of sport takes us back to "the Tiger Woods Saga". Sport has now become a powerful social institution exerting influence for the betterment of society. Then, all of a sudden, a "sport hero" of the highest magnitude behaves himself in such a way that basic societal values are challenged. Hence, we now must ask ourselves: "Specifically what are *the* values that Tiger has forsaken that have occasioned this world-wide outburst of publicity"?

"Socio-Instrumental" (Material) Values or "Moral" (Non-Material) Values?

Examining this matter carefully, we may be surprised to learn that sport's contribution to human wellbeing is a highly complicated matter. On the one side, there are those who claim that sport contributes significantly to the development of what are regarded as the *socio-instrumental* values--that is, the values of teamwork, loyalty, self-sacrifice, aggressiveness, and perseverance consonant with prevailing corporate capitalism in democracy and in most other political systems as well. In the process of making this "contribution," however, we discover also that there is now a good deal of evidence that in the process of contributing to the "global ideal" of capitalism, democracy, and advancing technology, sport has developed an ideal that opposes the historical, fundamental *moral* values of honesty, fairness, good will, sportsmanship, and responsibility in the innumerable competitive experiences provided (Lumpkin, Stoll, and Beller, 1999).

Significant to this discussion are the results of investigations carried out by Hahm, Stoll, Beller, Rudd, and others in recent years. The Hahm-Beller Choice Inventory (HBVCI) has now been administered to athletes at different levels in a variety of venues. It demonstrates conclusively that athletes are increasingly *not* supporting what is considered "the moral ideal" in competition. As Stoll and Beller (1998) reported, for example, an athlete with moral character demonstrates the moral character traits of honesty, fair play, respect, and responsibility whether an official is present to enforce the rules or not. (Priest, Krause, and Beach substantiated this finding in 1999). They reported that changes over a four-year period in a college athlete's ethical value choices were consistent with other investigations. Their findings showed *decreases* in "sportsmanship orientation" and an *increase* in "professional" attitudes associated with sport bespeaking so-called "social" values..

Aha! We have now arrived at the nub of the matter! Alas for poor Tiger Woods… His plight is that he is "caught" right in the middle of this ongoing controversy about the presumed contribution of sport. No matter which way he turns, he is "out of step" with the claims for sport made by either group. His actions clash with those who say that sport contributes to *instrumental* values. In addition, they also clash with those who argue that sport contributes to *moral* values. The perennial winner in golf, poor Tiger can't win now for losing! On the one hand he has confounded those who argue for "the instrumental–values contribution", and–on the other hand–he has betrayed those who promote sport because it makes "a moral-values contribution". Hence, many of his advertisers are now deserting Tiger because his commercial value to them has been tarnished perhaps irrevocably. The gross stock value of a number of his sponsors has decreased appreciably since Tiger has been exposed. Concurrently, the sports *hero*, that staunch fellow presumably with all of those fine moral values, has betrayed his fans young and old because of his "nocturnal peregrinations." Woe is Tiger!

Concluding Statement

Even though dictionaries define *social* character similarly, many sport practitioners, including participants, coaches, parents, and officials, have gradually come to believe that character is defined properly by such values as self-sacrifice, teamwork, loyalty, and perseverance. The common expression in competitive sport is: "He or she showed character"--meaning

"He/she 'hung in there' to the bitter end!" [or whatever...]. Rudd (1999) confirmed that coaches explained character as "work ethic and commitment." This coincides with what sport sociologists have found. Sage (1998. p. 614) explained: "Mottoes and slogans such as 'sports builds character' must be seen in the light of their ideological issues." In other words, competitive sport is structured by the nature of the society in which it occurs. This would appear to mean that over-commercialization, drug-taking, cheating, bribe-taking by officials, violence, etc. at all levels of sport are simply reflections of the culture in which we live.

Robert Osterhoudt (2010), one of the world's leading sport philosophers, offers a fundamental distinction to this troubling development as follows:

> . . . it does seem to me as well that such social values as earnest effort, dedication, self-sacrifice, and the like are meaningfully talked about in respect to sport and become defensible features of it *only if* they occur in the service of sport's inherent character as playful, competitive, and physical, not if they occur in the service of other forms of aim, such as commercial, nationalist, or military aim in particular. *The most fundamental distinction in all of this is thus the dividing of intrinsic and instrumental values, not the dividing of moral and social values.* (This is so because moral values, as described, serve *inherently*, thus becoming distinctly human ends.)

Where does all of this leave us today as we consider sport's presumed relationship with both *moral* character development and with *socio-instrumental* character development? Whatever your conclusion may be, Tiger Woods has been unexpectedly trapped in this "socio-instrumental" versus "moral" character vise that characterizes sport participation at the beginning of the 21st century. He tried to have it both ways. For his and his family's sake, let us hope that he will learn from this tragic experience—and that "the world" will "forgive his sins"...

References

Hahm, C.H., Beller, J. M., & Stoll, S. K. (1989). *The Hahm-Beller Values Choice Inventory*. Moscow, Idaho: Center for Ethics, The University of Idaho.

Lumpkin, A., Stoll, S., & Beller, J. M. (1999). *Sport ethics: Applications for fair play* (2nd ed.). St. Louis, MO: McGraw-Hill.

Marx, L. (1990). Does improved technology mean progress? In Teich, A. H. (Ed.), *Technology and the future*. NY: St. Martin's Press.

Osterhoudt, R. G. (2010). Personal correspondence, April 9. For a further insightful analysis of the situation, see Osterhoudt's "Concluding Postscript" (pp. 723-726) in Osterhoudt's *Sport as a form of human fulfillmentÚ An organic philosophy of sport history* (Victoria, BC, Canada, 2006)

Priest, R. F., Krause, J. V., & Beach, J. (1999). Four-year changes in college athlctcs' cthical valuc choiccs in sports situations. *Research Quarterly for Exercise and Sport,* 70(1), 170-178.

Rudd, A., Stoll, S. K., & Beller, J. M. (1999). Measuring moral and social character among a group of Division 1A college athletes, non-athletes, and ROTC military students. *Research Quarterly for Exercise and Sport,* 70 (Suppl. 1), 127.

Sage, G. H. (1998). Sports participation as a builder of character? *The World and I*, 3, 629-641.

Stoll, S. K. & Beller, J. M. (1998). *Sport as education: On the edge*. NY: Columbia University Teachers College.

Wilcox, R. C. (1991). Sport and national character: An empirical analysis. *Journal of Comparative Physical Education and Sport.*, XIII(1), 3-27.

Chapter 9
What Price Sport Heroes?

Big league baseball muddles along toward its annual tiresome reincarnation. The endless hockey season moves on to the eventual real games of the play-offs. One or the other brand of football--the North American kind or that which the rest of the world plays--can be called up on the tv screen at just about any hour of the day.

Everything considered, we are fortunate, but also sad, that the scourge of amytrophic lateral sclerosis (ALS) was needed to help Americans remember Lou Gehrig! And we are also relieved that hockey has given North America a Wayne Gretzky! However, we must admit that true sport heroes have been in short supply in recent years.

A Shortage of Mythical Heroes in America

Writing about mythical heroes in the U.S.A., R. Kahn stated: "There is an appalling shortage of genuine myth in this country's background. There are semi-myth figures such as Washington, minor-myth figures such as Paul Bunyan, nonsense-myth figures such as Superman, but there is no Roland, no Arthur, no Siegfried. Obligingly and profitably, sports promoters have thrown their hirelings into the breach." Kahn was arguing was that Hollywood offered us Marilyn Monroe as Aphrodite, and that sport gave us Babe Ruth as Zeus. Yuck!

Let's get down to specifics. A hero has been defined as "a man or woman of distinguished courage or ability admired for brave deeds and noble qualities," whereas a culture hero is explained as "a mythicized historical figure who embodies the aspirations or ideals of a society." Transferring these thoughts to sport, there is no doubt but that people really do believe that Babe Ruth was the United States sport hero of the 20th century. (In Canada the outstanding athlete of the first half century was Lionel Conacher.)

In addition, the U.S. has mistakenly elevated "the Babe" to the status of *culture hero* as well. Further, such adulation has extended mistakenly down to the present day, since Hofstra University, Long Island, NY, actually held a symposium honoring the 100th anniversary of the birth of "The Sultan of Swat." How ridiculous can these folks be?

A Wrongly Chosen Culture Hero!

Conversely, through a sin of omission, as I see it, the United States rates much lower--to a most significant degree--another outstanding professional athlete on the same team who contributed at least equally to the team's win-loss record in those glory years. The late Lou Gehrig--who is at least remembered today because a terrible disease is popularly named after him--made his accomplishments in a quiet, unassuming, gentlemanly, and sportsmanlike manner. Imagine this: in a survey of 31 sport historians, 29 of the group selected Ruth as the greatest sport figure in American history. Thus, whereas Ruth ranked first, Gehrig ranked 28 of the 31 sport figures who were named.

I was forced to ask myself how this could happen in a country with the espoused values and ideals of the United States. Just think about U.S. history and the people whose memories have been cherished. Now, answer this series of questions keeping these two athletes in mind.

Who came from a poor background and yet worked his way through college? (Of course, as did Gehrig, Ruth came from a very poor background.)

Who was a ruggedly handsome young man?

Who was shy and modest? (At least Hollywood picked Gary Cooper, and not William Bendix, to play Gehrig's part in a terrible movie.)

Who neither drank nor chased women, and who never broke curfew?

Who was characterized by Ty Cobb as "the hustlinest ball player I ever saw." (This was no mean compliment coming from one who probably deserved that accolade himself!)

And the list of questions continues. . . .

Who practiced unbelievably hard to correct his fielding deficiencies at first base?

Who took care of his poor, old mother on the way up (actually, the lady was the cook/maid at his Columbia University fraternity house)?

Who batted in the clean-up (No. 4) spot in the line-up of the "mighty Yankees?"

Who forced opposing pitchers to pitch to Babe Ruth (who was batter No. 3), rather than walk him) because they knew they would be facing Gehrig next?

Who matched Ruth homer for homer right down to the wire in that year (and ended up with 47 himself) when Ruth established his record of 60 home runs?

Who played 2,130 consecutive, complete baseball games for 14 consecutive years despite "beanings, fractures of toes and fingers, fevers, torn tendons, sprained ankles, pulled muscles, lumbago, colds, and other mishaps" (Gallico, 1942)?

Finally, and this list of questions could be extended even further, who--despite Ruth's home-run accomplishment that year--was voted the most valuable player in the American League by the sportswriters in that same year of 1927? The answer to all of these questions is *Lou Gehrig*!

I can come to no other conclusion: Lou Gehrig, the Babe's teammate, is actually the person who should have been named as the greatest sportsman--a culture hero, in fact--and this recognition should have carried through down to the present.

Crepeau in writing about the "tensions of the twenties" viewed this decade "as an important watershed in the development of the United States." In commenting about George Herman Ruth, he stated that "Ruth is the essence of the rugged individual playing the national game of the cow pasture in an urban stadium before the cheering masses of the machine age."

America Has an Idealistic Superstructure And a Materialistic Base

Building on this statement that seems to epitomize the early 20th century growth of the world's largest and most powerful capitalistic democracy, it becomes understandable why a number of philosophers and other critics have argued that the United States has had "an idealistic superstructure and a materialistic base!" If this be true, it is probably nowhere more evident than in the way that Babe Ruth and Lou Gehrig, two of the more important "elements" who made up the "Pride of the Yankees," have been evaluated by sport historians and most citizens in the States then and down to the present.

"The Babe" has become a culture hero of the greatest magnitude despite the very obvious, serious flaws in his character, while "Larrupin' Lou," Ruth's teammate, is only remembered fondly by some baseball aficionados as an excellent durable athlete with many fine personality traits (and, of course, also by those who know what amytrophic lateral sclerosis is!)

What we have here, I maintain, is a situation where history has given a much higher rating to an outstanding professional athlete who possessed a disproportionate amount of arrogance and flair for the dramatic, traits that were coupled with other character flaws that seemingly flaunted the avowed values of the nation. Whereas it (history) rates much lower--to a most significant degree--another outstanding professional athlete on the same team who contributed at least equally to the Yankees' success in those glory years, but who did it in a quiet, unassuming, gentlemanly, and sportsmanlike manner. If this assessment of the situation is correct, what does it tell us about athletes and highly competitive sport in our culture? Also, if this assessment of the situation is correct, what does this tell us about the United States and its millions of sports fans?

Question: Is Sport a Socially Useful Servant?

Was sport a "socially useful servant" then, and can it still be regarded as such today? If the answer is that sport is not really an important, useful social force today, what good is it anyhow? Is it enough, for example, for sport to serve as entertainment or an escape from daily responsibilities--the "opiate of the masses"? Further, why do we condone today--or at least "look the other way" when they occur--i.e., some of the shameful and often illegal actions of athletes, and then turn right around and condemn severely similar behavior by non-athletes in everyday life?

This is a highly important matter about which intelligent, influential people must become increasingly concerned. Competitive sport has steadily increased in importance as a social force in the world, exerting almost too great an influence if this is possible. We simply cannot continue to look the other way at the daily misconduct that is reported on the part of spectators, athletes, coaches, and administrators in professional, semiprofessional, and amateur sport.

Further, culture heroes are truly hard to come by these days. If we really want America to be among the finest of nations in all regards, and if we really feel that sport has an important contribution to make to the development of such a society, I believe it is time to give the highest reward and acclaim to whose who demonstrate through sport both a high degree of athletic ability *and* the finest of personality and character traits.

If we were functioning according to such criteria, it would be Gehrig who is the folk hero today, and Ruth who is remembered as the "home run king" with the badly flawed character and personality. These characterizations are simply not clear in the minds of most citizens, young or old.

I can only conclude that times are indeed changing--for the worse. Whereas at various times throughout history, the world had its Hercules, Samson, Beowulf, and Siegfried, it was concluded recently that, in western culture, Stallone (as Rocky or Rambo?) has served to reinforce our conception of the heroes who emerged in recent years.

One social analyst (S.D. Stark, 1987) reacted to a world where society had lost control and thereby had failed its citizens. He stated, "Many scholars, for example, place Mr. Stallone--and let's not forget Mr. Schwarzenegger who couldn't take time off from body building to attend his father's funeral--squarely in the footsteps of John Wayne and Clint Eastwood. He says his heroes display much of "the same rugged, macho individualism as the old heroes of westerns . . ."

American Heroes Are Chosen Irrationally

People need to understand through use of their own rational powers that they are being increasingly lured or marketed daily by others into reactions dominated more by emotions than reason. It may well be necessary to reinforce individual ego at the various geographic and social levels (i.e. community, region, state or province, nation) by the creation of heroes and heroines in the various aspects of social living (including sport). To what extent this should be done through the artificial creation of Superman, Wonderwoman, Spiderman, Rambo, and Indiana Jones is debatable. However, it may somehow serve a beneficial purpose when such individuals do not appear normally in the course of ongoing events.

Further, if this type of aggrandizement (self- or promoter-sponsored) is what is happening in competitive sport, we might ask to what extent highly competitive sport is indeed a "socially useful servant" today? We know how difficult it is to make a case for the building of desirable character and personality traits through the medium of sport. Nevertheless should our values become so perverted that we condone certain unsportsmanlike and illegal actions in sport and athletics at any level.

Intelligent, influential people must become very concerned about this anomaly in social life. If we really believe that sport has an important contribution to make to the development of a fine society, is it not time to give the highest reward and acclaim to whose who demonstrate through sport both a high degree of athletic ability and the finest of personality and character traits?

America Should Separate True Heroes from Celebrities

We should give high priority to bringing about a change in the present state of affairs as soon as possible. An important responsibility of those involved with sport in a truly professional manner should be to help people separate the true heroes and heroines from the celebrities. This might help to offset the condition prevailing in which the media offer us the "packaged hero" for consumption.

In 1975 Fishwick told us that the hero is a reflection of the place and the era in which he lives. Accordingly, despite the fact that the media needs celebrity figures to sell their wares, and despite the fact that politicians need a variety of symbols that are somehow supposed to reflect glory on them, the people themselves must insist that heroes and heroines, in sport or any other aspect of life, truly reflect the finest societal values that we proclaim for our culture.

London in 1978 stated, "The hero is an extinct species relegated to the memory of my youthful idealism . . . This is the age of the superstar, not the hero. And superstars specialize in self-adulation, not sacrifice." Lou Gehrig did not specialize in self-adulation; neither did Terry Fox, nor does Wayne Gretzky nor Silken Laumann for that matter do so today. In one of her well-known songs, Peggy Lee said it all with one plaintive question--presumably not thinking of competitive sport--"Is that all there is?"

If people such as Gehrig and Gretzky are continually held up as role models and truly given the type of recognition they deserve, we would be in a much better position to argue logically that highly competitive sport is indeed an important useful social force. However, if we continue to condone (as we often look the other way) distasteful, unsportsmanlike, overly mercenary actions in sport, we are simply affirming the negative aspects of sport as an entertainment device in an otherwise (presumably) boring existence.

Chapter 10
The Use of Power by Coaches and Officials in Competitive Sport

"We have faults which we have hardly used yet," said Pogo, the cartoon character created by Walt Kelley. This typically wise creature could easily have been describing the current situation in society where a great variety of contemporary villains continue to affect the quality of life of our lives both directly and indirectly. I'm referring here to shoplifters, crooked politicians, liars, tax evaders, white-collar shysters, violent criminals, vandals, expense-account "padders," pimps, economic exploiters, wife-abusers, petty thieves, bullies of one sort or another, and so forth.

What categories have I forgotten? No matter; for our present discussion you get the message. With such a situation prevailing to varying degrees in Canada, the United states, and Mexico, we can only speculate whether it is better or worse anywhere else in the world. With such a situation prevailing, and I am really not trying to be especially pessimistic, we can hardly expect that competitive sport would be free from society's influences. Or, conversely, to our great chagrin, we are rapidly becoming able to ask to what extent the growing negative influences from sport are affecting societal life.

I'll let you be the judge. Every ten years or so during my career of close to 60 years, I have assessed the ethical situation in competitive sport, that presumably great character-building agency that we all love. These past analyses were typically discouraging, to put it mildly. You may ask, "That was then~ what about the situation today?" I wish I could report that conditions had improved, but this is just not the case. In fact, the situation has, if anything, worsened. And, sadly, what was reported in each of my earlier limited investigations was just the tip of the iceberg.

The Current Situation in Society and Sport

Maybe we have become inured to such reports, and we just don't pay as much attention as we did formerly (another "Royal Commission," so to speak). At any rate, the series of incidents I recently collected at random taken from *The New York Times* (unless indicated otherwise), began in late 1995 and ended with the "bite of the century" in mid-1997. Because of the subjective nature of much of this information, as was the case with my earlier "look-sees," no direct comparative evaluation is possible. However, the situation is evidently as bad as ever, and it may indeed be growing worse steadily. Consider the following:

1. In an article titled "Not sweet, and not a science," Barry (Nov. 26, 1995) reported the growing popularity of a new sport called extreme or ultimate fighting. The activity resembles video games such as "Mortal Kombat" that feature bare-knuckled encounters between fighters who can punch and kick with abandon while obeying only one cardinal rule: no eye-gouging!

2. More than 20 years after the U.S. Congress decided that opportunities for men and women to take part in intercollegiate athletics must be equal, the U.S. Education Department has published a new set of rules requiring colleges and universities to make annual reports on expenditures available for both men's and women's intercollegiate athletics (Dec. 3, 1995). This was deemed necessary since many of these institutions were still not complying with Title IX legislation enacted in the 1970s. (This was an act requiring equal treatment for both sexes).

3. The "Great Snowball Bombing" (Berkow, Dec. 28, 1995) related an incident that took place on Dec. 23 in which literally thousands of fans at a football game first took to throwing snowballs at each other, but eventually switched to throwing them at the people on the playing field with resultant injuries. As a result 75 people were barred for life from the stadium, and charges were filed against one spectator who could be identified from a newspaper photo••

4. The following day (Dec. 29, 1995), Allen Barra's piece "Sentenced to play football" reviewed the Phillips case at the University of Nebraska in September, an incident in which this football star battered his girlfriend to the floor in her apartment and then dragged her down three flights of stairs to the street. His arrest and subsequent suspension from the team ended after he had missed six games and the University

"sentenced" him to "mandatory counseling, community service, and attendance at all classes."

5. After a century in which many institutions of higher education in the United states have been "dogs wagged by athletic tails," an editorial (Jan. 23, 1996) stated that "The N.C.A.A. Gets It Right." This editorial celebrates the fact that--"after a 10-year power struggle within the National collegiate Athletic Association--the group that sets rules for undergraduate sports--college presidents have won a big victory in their campaign to control runaway athletic programs." Of course, this doesn't mean that the battle has been won; in fact, it is just beginning on the basis of a more level battlefield! At any rate, the editorial concluded: "The presidents will need energy, courage and their trustees if the effort is to succeed." Don't bet on their success…

6. Moving from the general to a more specific item, on February 2, 1996 the Times described a case at Virginia Polytechnic and state University in which a first-year student there claimed that she was raped by two freshman football players in her dormitory. The University's evident lax approach to the incident has occasioned a ground-breaking lawsuit against the two athletes and the University. This has become a civil rights issue under the 1994 Violence Against Women Act.

7. Mixed in with this litany of unsavory practices relating to sport was one lone heartening article by Larry Dorman (March 20, 1996). Stated he, "If we need any further evidence that golf is an oasis of integrity in a sports desert of mendacity, it came this past weekend." This startling event was Jeff Sluman's disqualification of himself from the Bay Hill Invitational Gold Tournament. Why had he done so? He did this simply because he believed, but was not certain, that he had broken a tournament rule the day before by taking an improper drop (in this case retrieving his ball from the water and dropping it in a so-called drop zone). The reason for the inclusion of this item is simply that deliberate living up to a rule in sport especially when not being observed--or even the

99

spirit of the rule, is such an anachronism today that it simply had to be featured in the country's leading newspaper!

8. Moving to a different sub-topic within sport ethics, Hank Aaron (April 13, 1997), writing on the 50th anniversary of the first Black's admission to the major leagues--and telling about a man he saw as a hero (Jackie Robinson)--decried the prevailing spirit of sport: a lust for money. Stated Aaron, "The result is that today's players have lost all concept of history. Their collective mission is greed. Nothing else means much of anything to them. As a group, there's no discernible social conscience among them; certainly no sense of self-sacrifice, which is what Jackie Robsinson's legacy is based on... People wonder where the heroes have gone. Where there is no conscience, there are no heroes" (E, 15).

9. One month later, in a "special report": titled "Over the edge," Bamberger and Yaeger (SI, April 14, 1997) presented the essence of a study carried out with 198 Olympians. One hundred and ninety-five of 198 surveyed stated that they would take illegal, performance-enhancing substances if they were guaranteed that (1) they would not be caught, and (2) they would win. When the guarantee of winning and not being caught was extended to a period of five years, with the added proviso that the athlete would die from the side effects of the drug consumed, 50% stated that they would take it nevertheless. The authors concluded that the availability of literally hundreds of substances has caused athletes, "aware that drug testing is a sham," to "seem to rely more than ever on banned performance enhancers" (p. 61).

10. In a second article in the same issue of ax titled "Under suspicion," Bamberger related the tale of one swimmer from Ireland named Michelle Smith. The author argued that, "after winning three gold medals in Atlanta, Michelle Smith should be a big star--but too many people believe that her victories were drug-aided" (p. 73). The suspicion is that at age 26 her accomplishments were literally incredible because "most female swimmers are a half decade beyond their best

performances" (p. 74). Ms. Smith claims that she is drug-free. If this is true, her "social" ostracism is a real tragedy.

This capsule updating of "the situation" in competitive sport must end with no. 10 again. Skipping over another report that Title IX in the US. has not leveled the playing field (June 16, 1997, p. 1), we find a column by Latham Forbes in Toronto's *The Globe and Mail* (May 2, 1997, p. A22) characterizes hockey as being "about macho goons and raging egos in all their tough-guys-don't-dance glory"; a "BackTalk" column (June 29, 1997, "Sports, II p. 19) that stresses the fact that far too often screaming adults (typically parents) are taking all the fun out of playing for Little Leaguers; a humorous piece by the irreverent Russell Baker titled "Sport marches on" (Nov. 9, 1996) that ridicules the prevailing "sport mentality" (e.g., "Humbert Ballew, onetime star defensive end for the Washington Thickskins, has revealed that hc is using his retirement years learning to read"); and, finally, Harvey Araton's column "A misguided and warped value system" (June 28, 1997) that chronicles Lefkowitz's description of the 1989 rape case in which an "educable mentally retarded" girl was sexually assaulted by a group of popular high school athletes.

Finally, we come to Joyce Carol Oates's "Fury and fine lines" (July 3, 1997) that discusses what has been facetiously been labeled "the bite of the century" mentioned above. This action, which actually should have been described as plural (bites!), was executed twice in frustration by Mike Tyson in his heavyweight championship fight with Evander Holyfield. In this horrible activity, labeled as sport by some, Ms. Oates wrote that "Mike Tyson, it's now clear," was not" "inspired to fight bravely and more dangerously than before" " (p. AlS). Ms. Oates declared that in his (incisive!) action "Tyson has provided us with an iconic moment." So be it; the sporting world marches on.

A Growing Interest in Ethics and Morality

Seemingly endless incidents such as these take us into the realm of ethics and morality, a topic that is receiving an increasingly greater amount of attention in professional preparation in many fields today. We are discovering, however, that the entire matter is quite thoroughly tangled. Somehow we find ourselves tied into knots from which we are only feebly seeking to extricate ourselves. And nowhere do we seem to find weaker efforts to escape from our ethical dilemma than in the realm of highly competitive sport. We hope that the "good guys" will win, but we are haunted by the slogan that "nice guys finish last"--and who wants to be a "good loser?"

Part of our problem stems from the fact that, in this stage of so-called postmodern civilization in North America, there is no longer one major ethical tradition. How the many different strands of ethical tradition from around the world have been woven into a variety of ethical patterns, thus creating an amalgam of often conflicting values and norms. This has made it highly difficult, if not impossible, for one ethical credo to emerge. Often the lowest common denominator prevails.

Thus, today we have been influenced by (1) the Hebraic culture based on the Ten Commandments; (2) the Christian system based on the Beatitudes, (3) the Medieval way of life based on penance; (4) the Renaissance culture based on individual development along with freedom; (5) the Industrial Revolution based on the application of science to technology; (6) the scientific approach based on empirical method and its influence on the determination of truth; (7) the impact of a multi-ethnic culture with the influence of the various, ever-present religious creeds in the background; and, finally, (8) the prevailing confusion because we are presumably leaving the modern period behind to cross the "post-modern divide" as we lunge into the 21st century.

Our dilemma today, rather than continuing along as at present seemingly hopelessly mired in the sludge that characterizes the welter of conflicting value systems that prevail, is to seek to make change within a situation that demands our most serious attention. Professional sport is not going to lead us to the "promised land"; that's for certain. More is the current "Olympic mentality" going to guide us in the right direction either. How can we differentiate between it and what the pros" are doing? I say to you people here today that sport, if it is to truly be a "socially useful" influence, will have to be gradually made so by men and women of enlightened good will in Canada--people such as you obviously are as demonstrated by your attendance at these sessions--who will do it through the medium of competitive sport that is ~to our highest ideals for humanity!

The Demand for Improved Levels of Performance

The entire problem of drugs and performance is one that demands continuing investigation. Of course, this is only part of a still 6 greater societal issue. And it is true, of course, that many different natural and synthetic chemical substances and preparations have been used since ancient times in an effort to improve endurance and subsequent physical performance. Our concern is obviously to make sense of it all because stimulants, painkillers, and other body-building agents are being employed by athletes to a greater or lesser extent. We, as coaches, officials, athletic therapists, sport psychologists and physiologists, and administrators, are in a position to monitor and control this situation to a degree by vigorously promoting the idea of "fair play," a concept called for a generation ago by Peter McIntosh (1979).

Just how many people of all ages have been, and are presently, involved with the consumption of some type of stimulants, painkillers, and "bodybuilders" as part of their efforts toward winning and high-level achievement in competitive sport? How is such consumption hurting these people physically and psychologically? Who knows? One can't help but believe, however, that this problem has assumed large proportions, and that its severity is increasing almost daily. Who will not agree that we are going to hear more, rather than less, about this perplexing and vexing problem in the months and years ahead?

Coach and Athlete: In Each Other's Power

The scenario has now been outlined. We now have a hypothesized chain of events in which one person may be exploited or used by another. I suppose it could be argued that it is usually the coach who exploits the athlete, but I can also argue that sometimes the opposite is the case. Also, interestingly, there is a third possibility: that the athlete is presumably exploiting himself or herself when he or she "enters the drug scene."

Permit me to insert a personal note here. I came to Canada from the United States twice (in 1949 and in 1971), the second time to stay and become a citizen. One of the main reasons for this was my inability to cope psychologically with the effects of "big-time" intercollegiate athletics in the states. The power being exerted, the entrapment taking place with no noticeable effects on the consciences of the coaches or others involved, and the everyday exploitation of young men ("my kids," as coaches are wont to say about their post-21 year behemoth charges), not to mention the humiliation to those of us engaged professionally in physical education and educational sport striving to maintain academic standards, began to literally make me ill. So, in a sense, I "retreated" to Canada where I could breathe the almost pure air of competitive sport again (except for "the Cross" we bear with professional hockey!). In the process I was now able in good conscience once again to cheer for our teams at Western Ontario and to appreciate that the athletes on our teams were, very largely, student-athletes. Also, no longer did I, as an administrator, have to say: "We in physical education really don't have any problems with intercollegiate sport; they're over there on the other side of the campus."

Let us consider first, then, the situation in which the athlete may be exploited by the coach. For example, you may be familiar with the late-1970s situation in California in which a number of athletes sued the coach and a university because they had presumably been used. They had been brought to the university with the lure of athletic scholarships, university degrees, and perhaps an opportunity to play "pro ball." However, in the final analysis, they argued, specific "academic" programs were recommended so that continuing eligibility would be maintained, and also a trust had been broken because the desired educational knowledge and competency was not acquired. In many cases, not even the academic degree was obtained either, and the athletes were "cast adrift" because eligibility had been used up after four years of play. Finally, to make the case even stronger, let us imagine something that we do not actually know--that during the time of active participation, the athletes were often encouraged to take certain illegal stimulants, painkillers, and body-building agents. Certainly this final stipulation is well within the realm of possibility and is probably occurring regularly in the case of many male--and now female too!--athletes within a variety of sports in the United States and elsewhere around the world.

The situation just described brings us face to face with a philosophical--if not a legal--question to which we may seek appropriate and just answers. Am I morally forbidden to treat a person entirely as a means to some other end? The "greatest good for the greatest number" argument of the utilitarians (Mill) does seemingly give us the opportunity to use a person to some extent for the good of the whole. Further, it can be argued that a Kantian ~pursue the greatest good while only viewing the welfare of an individual involved as a "side constraint" while in active pursuit of a higher goal or greater good.

Another interesting question is whether it is wrong to use a person even though the individual concerned doesn't believe that she or he has been wronged and is actually quite happy about the involvement. Such use of a person may also been described as deception, and is thus wrong any way one looks at it. If the individual being used is not actually deceived, then such use is a separate wrong.

Definitions

As we continue this discussion, please keep these definitions in mind:

Power is defined as "the ability or official capacity to exercise control or influence over another."

Deception is an act by which a person is misled as to the actual state of affairs.

Entrapment is the "actions that lure another into danger, difficulty, or self-incrimination"; "is thus a form of treachery, an abuse of trust."

Exploitation (which usually accompanies entrapment) is the "utilization of another for selfish purposes"; thus, if entrapment is the treacherous acquisition of power over a person, exploitation is using such power for selfish ends." (See Wilson, 1978, p. 303.)

To continue, if entrapment involves the treacherous acquisition of power gained possibly through deception, and exploitation is the use of such power for selfish ends, these are obviously general questions of a moral nature that arise when any form of official or unofficial power is employed. This would be true if those ends are either selfish or benevolent. Why is this so? It is true because the source of power serves as a lever by which one individual can move another person to do this or not to do that. Now it becomes obvious to us as coaches and teachers what a tremendous ethical responsibility we have in our everyday dealings with athletes. Think about it;

isn't this a responsibility that often appears to have been assumed in an almost unbelievably light manner? Of course, as we stated above, the basic philosophical question that arises here throughout this discussion is whether we morally forbidden to treat another person as a means to some other end?

The Sources of Interpersonal Power

Who holds such power, "the ability or official capacity to exercise control or influence over others?" Politicians have such power or influence; bureaucrats have it; CEOs in the business world have it; parents have it; and coaches and officials most certainly have such power to influence their typically eager charges. our basic concern here, of course, is the power or leverage that the coach can exert for good or bad (e.g., the leverage that he/she can apply in regard to whether the athlete takes stimulants, painkillers, or body-building agents regularly to improve performance and thereby to achieve greater success for himself or herself and for the coach involved). The position of the official is similar, but from a different perspective.

What are these elements or sources of interpersonal power (held primarily by the coach) that may be brought to bear on aspiring athletes, elements that must be employed very carefully and with foresight because of the great impact they may have? First, the concept of "love" is perhaps the major one of a number of similar feelings that one person might have for another. other terms to describe such a feeling are affection, respect, awe, friendship, admiration, and trust. If an athlete has any or all of these feelings for his/her coach, the coach is then continually faced with an assessment of what constitutes a reasonable request that might be made of the athlete--and what might actually be an imposition. If the coach were to make too great a demand of the athlete based on the amount of love or similar emotion felt, the reaping of excess benefit from such an excessive demand could well constitute exploitation to a greater or lesser extent. Also, in the case of the athlete, other feelings that might accompany those mentioned above would be gratitude, indebtedness, obligation, and desire for approval. (For use of these terms in another context, see Wilson, 1978, pp. 304-307.)

Second, a frequent source of power over another that is held by the coach is that of fear--fear that can be overt, subtle, and is often irrational. A coach has a powerful lever here that can be used with an athlete if and when deemed necessary. The athlete may be afraid of losing his/her salary, honorarium, award, scholarship, education, place on the team, status as an athlete (including possible future employment), and even status as a person.

A third source of interpersonal power that could well place the coach in too strong a position vis a vis the athlete is that the athlete may have too strong a desire, or too pressing a need, to make the grade athletically. A coach does not have to be exceptionally bright to understand this, and therefore may be tempted occasionally to use such a desire or need for his/her own end--even if such use were against the best interests of the athlete concerned. (Many athletes, in America especially, come from so-called lower-middle and lower economic classes; so, there may well be an urgent need, and therefore a stronger desire, to "make it" both financially and socially in the society.)

A fourth way that is open to a selfish or unscrupulous person in our society, one whereby an advantage of another individual may be taken, is through the exploitation of that person's virtues or qualities of character. In competitive sport a greedy, unscrupulous coach can quite easily exploit such qualities of the athlete as tolerance, good manners, goodness of nature, gentleness, unselfishness, and sense of responsibility.

By turning the "virtue coin" over, we immediately discover a fifth mechanism--that of character defects--that may be employed by person A to gain power over person B. The athlete may be gullible, susceptible to flattery, foolhardy, vain, or may also be easily subject to feelings of dislike and even hatred of a particular team or opponent. Such emotions are often very easily triggered by an unthinking or possibly unethical coach.

How we can turn that virtue-vice coin over once again, because down through the ages youth has been especially prone to idealistic, unselfish commitments to worthwhile causes. Such willingness to pledge allegiance may take the form of love of, or pride in, or concern for another. This sixth mechanism that might be used by a coach appeals to such elements as loyalty, idealism, patriotism, etc. For the athlete this involves a commitment, at times irrational, to someone or something outside of himself or herself.

A seventh mechanism often exercised to gain power over another person is that of knowledge. How often have we heard the phrase "knowledge is power" in recent years? How we are told almost daily that the ignorant, naive, and inexperienced person is practically powerless in our society in relation to those people who have the facts and know-how to put them to work. In the case of the athlete, the coach and his associates usually know a great deal more about life itself and the sport in which the young person is taking part. In fact, typically a disproportionate mystique is built up around such knowledge, knowledge that quite often lacks a scientific base. Nevertheless, the young athlete usually puts his or her trust in the coach and will typically follow their directions in just about all matters. It would there seem to make sense that the coach should periodically review just what responsibilities go along with the holding of such knowledge and resultant power.

An eighth consideration for the coach, or any person in society relating to another for that matter, is the situation in which A finds B rendered relatively powerless because of some temporary or permanent handicap or incapacity. Such a condition could easily be exploited by a coach who is presumably in possession of all his/her faculties. In fact, the coach could well be more intelligent, more facile in thought and verbal capacity, and more self-confident. Thus, the injured athlete, the student with a questionable academic record, or the person lacking self-confidence (for one of a variety of reasons) could well be dominated by an unscrupulous and/or thoughtless coach.

Finally, then, as ninth we can probably all agree that there will always be opportunities to exert power over others within a social system, because we will probably always find greater or lesser dependency existing in human relationships in any society that has been conceived to the present. This will be true with the status of a child, the aged, the infirm, the poor, the ignorant, the mentally handicapped, etc. In the case of the athlete, especially when there is financial subsidization that can be removed before the completion of an education, we typically find a great dependency on the coach. This dependency is present until graduation (a result that comes all too infrequently in many of these situations), until eligibility is used up, or until a pro contract is signed (a truly rare occurrence). (I should state parenthetically that I am in favor of the practice of striving for excellence in sport, as well as in other potentially "educational" experiences in campuses. And, if a bona fide student has proven financial need, I believe that he/she should receive financial assistance so that he/she can participate in these activities.

Summary and Conclusions

We began by stating that there is considerable evidence pointing to the conclusion that an increasing number of young men and women in various countries are consuming stimulants, painkillers, body-building agents, and endurance-building means. Despite prohibition by sports-governing bodies of over 400 of these substances, including temporary and/or permanent disqualification for those who are caught, the impossibility of testing everyone at all times for the possible use of so-called illegal substances is well known. Further, evidence is accumulating that temporary or permanent damage may result from their ingestion. Thus, we have a daily situation where the athlete, and his (or her) coach, are faced with fundamental ethical decisions in this regard.

Then we discussed the question of being in another person's power, a situation we all face in our own lives every day unless our name is Robinson Crusoe. Here, of course, this question was applied specifically to the relationship between coaches or officials and the athlete. The coach is therefore continually faced with ethical decisions as to when it is right to exercise certain levels of power so that good will result. If we join these two problems together, we can readily see that the athlete needs the finest type of guidance from this person, the coach or official, who has power over him or her.

As we have seen, power over another may be exercised for a number of different reasons: for one's own benefit; for the benefit of the other, for the shared benefit of oneself and the other, for the good of society, etc. We are brought to the conclusion finally that the coach truly faces an awesome responsibility today in this regard. The coach should be most careful not to rationalize using such power over an athlete for the coach's benefit by arguing that it is all right so long as the other is not hurt in some way or made unhappy thereby.

Finally, because of our heritage, and especially because we are being challenged on so many fronts in the world, we seem to be more concerned than ever before with the idea of success--of being *"Number One"* both materially and spiritually. This emphasis has accelerated to the point where it is fundamentally unhealthy and can be downright dangerous. Ratings, lists, polls, and other types of evaluation focus continually on *"Who"* or *"What"* is the *"Winner"*!

May I suggest that this so-called Lombardian ethic views success as winning, as a destination, rather than as one of a series of milestones along the way (i.e., only one of the journey). We might argue conversely and, I believe, rightly that there is only one destination in. life and that is death! What I am recommending coincides with the thought of Robert Louis

Stevenson: "To travel hopefully is a better thing than to arrive!" Such an aim about the ideal way to live explains that not everyone catches the brass ring on life's carousel. Most of us had better enjoy the ride for its own sake, or life could possibly have no true meaning at all. In the realm of sport, we as coaches should wield power intelligently with a social conscience in such a way that individuals lives are strengthened and enriched. The challenge we face is to make competitive sport into a beneficial social force that improves the society in which we live.

References

Araton, H. (1997). A misguided and warped value system. *The New York Times*, p. A36, June 28.

Aaron, H. (1997). When baseball mattered. *The New York Times*, p. E15, April 13.

Baker, R. (1997). Sports marches on. *The New York Times*, p. A17, Nov. 9.

Bamberger, M. (1997). Under suspicion. *Sports Illustrated*, 86, 15:73-85.

Bamberger, M. & Yaeger, D. (1997). Over the edge. *Sports Illustrated*, 86, 15:61-70.

Barra, A. (1995). Sentenced to play football. *The New York Times*, p. A11, Dec. 29.

Barry, D. (1995). Not sweet, and not a science. *The New York Times*, Sports, p. 11, Nov. 26.

Bernstein, N. (1996). civil rights lawsuit in rape case challenges integrity of a campus. *The New York Times*, p. 1, Feb. 11.

Berkow, I. (1995) The louts get their just reward from the Giants. *The New York Times*, p. B7, Dec. 28.

Chambers, M. (1997). For women, 25 years of Title IX has not leveled the playing field. *The New York Times*, pp. 1, C18, June 16.

Dorman, L. (1996). More than a drop of integrity for Sluman. *The New York Times*, p. 19, March 30.

Forbes, L. (1997). Macho goons or storied heroes? *The Globe and Mail* (Toronto), p. A22, May 2.

New York Times. The. (1996) The N.C.A.A. gets it right, p. A12, Jan. 23.

New York Times. The. (1997). Sports (Backtalk column), p. 19, June 29.

Oates, J.C. (1997). Fury and fine lines. *New York Times, The* A15, July 3.

Wilson, J.R.S. (July 1978). In one another's power. *Ethics*, 88, 4:299-315.

Chapter 11
America Is Screwing Up Competitive Sport

Note: This brief chapter was written after reading John Tirman's *100 Ways That America Is Screwing Up the World* (NY: Harper Perennial, 2006).

Why Have Sport?

Sport is being used increasingly to promote "instrumental" as opposed to "moral" values with the result that the whole ethos of sport within American culture has been transformed. This shift in the fundamental character of an increasingly popular activity within a society has now reached a point where you hear enlightened people asserting facetiously that "winning is not the most important thing any more: it's the *only* thing"!

Additionally it has been shown in studies that fair play, honesty, and sportsmanship actually decline steadily through athletes' university experience (Stoll, *et al.*). Further, this overemphasis on winning has been extended to international sport competition with a resultant increase in the taking of drugs and various supplements, an abuse that is well on its way to either make a mockery of highly competitive sport or "kill" it… Of course, this is all part and parcel of an "own the podium" mentality being promoted despite protests to the contrary by high-minded politicians and citizens.

This "own-the-podium" phrase has been adopted and supported financially by the Canadian government, for example, and who knows how many other government openly or surreptitiously? If this weren't bad enough, such occurrences have been accompanied by the fostering of a way of life that encourages "spectatoritis" in the general public instead of actual ongoing involvement in healthful physical activity and sport.

Sport Within Education

Within education, this overemphasis on winning has brought about a condition where infinitely more money is spent on varsity sport for the very few than is spent on intramural sports for the overwhelming majority of students. This is a situation that would shock education (and society!) to the core if it were allowed to happen to any other subject matter or activity sponsored within public education.

Such overemphasis has resulted in the development of so-called "tv sport universities" whose athletic efforts can be watched at almost any time on major networks or rented for view at additional cost on demand. Such programs are typically accompanied by 250-members marching bands and attractive, athletically oriented cheerleaders with typical prominent, jiggling body parts. It's a great show that brings the sponsoring university significant kudos with accompanying alumni financial support both legal and illegal... And don't let us forget the semi-professionalism of the athletes involved who may, *or quite often may not,* subsequently graduate with a bona fide degree from the institution attended.

The "Prevailing Mentality" Within Sport

Somehow I "understand," but don't think I'll every truly understand or appreciate the idea of "trash talk" in competitive sport that involves ongoing verbal abuse and slandering of opponents designed to cause them to play poorly. Or, for that matter, somehow I can't bring myself to approve of the "excessive showboating" by athletes when some phase of the activity at hand has been completed successfully.

However, I suppose this is only a minor problem when one considers aspects of sport like the ongoing brain damage that is permitted in professional boxing where there is no protective headgear for both men *and women).* Further, we are permitting (promoting?) the increasing development of "high-risk" sport where "life and limb" are increasingly threatened. Just think of parents going to court to get permission for their 12-yr. old child to sail around the world in a small boat alone to create a record...

Further, of course, we now have the privilege of paying to watch "all-out" combat (so-called "extreme sport") either in person or on television. In addition, to be fair to the feminine gender, women now have their own opportunities to perform for admiring sports fans in this "new" "sport."! Still further, I won't even mention what is termed professional wrestling, an activity that has long since departed from the realm of competitive *sport* (i.e., the winner has been determined in advance).

Mixed Martial Arts Is Abhorrent

Let me direct some of my harshest criticism to the whole idea of "martial-art" sport. It's "self-defense" that should be stressed- for children and young people, not aggression! As a former amateur wrestling coach and self-defense instructor training armed-forces personnel, I can only express my abhorrence to read that the "abomination" known as mixed-martial arts has been approved for professional performances in many venues in North America.

All young people–male (and female!)–should be taught self-defense in a complete program of physical activity education within pubic education. However, legalizing such aggressive activity as "martial arts" sends exactly the wrong message to youth. The promotion of outright, bestial aggressiveness for public display and vicarious involvement of spectators is inherently contradictory to the value system that I thought prevailed in North American society.

Already we can see the repercussions from the acceptance of such encounters. Youth across the country are trying it out with an assortment of arrangements in basements and schoolyards after school or at lunchtime. What's even worse is the addition of a female component to the (so-called) mixed-martial arts programs thereby only exacerbating the tone of the entire disgusting situation.

What could city council members be thinking of as they blithely give approval to these exhibitions portraying humans' inherent aggressive nature? They were probably too busy computing tax revenues to be accrued from the acceptance of this form of dubious entertainment for civic consumption. After all, their salaries need upward adjustment what with rising living costs…

A Few Final Thoughts

Permit me to offer a few final thoughts to what some "sportsmen and sportswomen" may already view as a diatribe. My first complaint relates to the paying ridiculously high salaries to professional athletes thus creating a "false sense of values" to youth and the older populace. In addition, the coach of football at one university earns makes well over two million dollars a year! Further, I simply cannot comprehend how a society could endorse these outrageous, multiyear contracts to a variety of coaches and athletes in the several gate-receipt sports. And, finally—if this isn't extreme enough—in Canada they recently named a lake after one athlete (a hockey player, of course), while at the same time a recommendation to name a comparable body of water after a *real* war hero was running into difficulty…

Chapter 12
Urgently Needed:
A Definition of Semi-Professionalism in Sport

A Confusing Situation

In North America during the 20th century we developed more than 100 different definitions of an amateur--but none of a semiprofessional!. This is why any attempt to define an amateur or a professional in sport correctly will soon bring you to a state where you begin to wonder whether you ever should have gotten involved.

Traditionally our brethren in the amateur sport organizations have described the amateur as follows:

> An amateur sportsperson is one who engages in
> sport solely for the pleasure and physical,
> mental, or moral benefits to be derived there-
> from and to whom sport is nothing more than
> an avocation.

Try explaining that definition to some of today's Olympic athletes in basketball and tennis!

Even a dictionary's innocuous statement that "an amateur is one who is not rated as a professional" leaves you high and dry. It helps a bit if you read further and learn that "a professional is one, generally, who has competed in athletics for a stake or purse, or gate money, or with a professional for a prize, or who has taught or trained in athletics for pay." But today this is now an outmoded definition. However, note that nowhere do we find an attempt to define a semiprofessional, a person for whom sport is presumably not the goal of a lifetime but more that of an avocation!

Finally--in desperation--you may agree that Paul Gallico had good insight when he stated many years ago, "An amateur is a guy who won't take a check!" Nowadays, however, even this formerly sage remark is a bit outdated. The international athlete may simply reply, "Please make it out to my trust fund after I have passed the drug test."

What Are the Characteristics of an Amateur?

Some go so far as to say that there are no more amateurs--at any level. This is not true. There are--and I hope there always will be--amateurs as defined in the traditional definition above. However, it is my hope that people like us will bring pressure to bear so that all will agree that the amateur is the beginner in any sphere of activity--including sport.

For example, when a young man or woman just learning the game of golf turns in a score of 125 for eighteen holes, he or she is indeed an amateur--a beginner or duffer in the game of golf. This coincides with the original meaning of the term "amateur" as "one who seeks to cultivate any art or pursuit for the enjoyment of it . . . sometimes implying desultory action or crude results." The amateur may simply lack the talent, desire, or polish of the semiprofessional or the professional.

From Amateurism to Semi–professionalism

If we think of the amateur as the beginner, the novice, the duffer (if you will), we might therefore argue that only sandlot or high school athletes are still amateur--and a relatively few college or university performers (notably in the Ivy League and in the Province of Ontario, Canada).

It would not be wrong to state, however, that semi–professionalism now abounds in many programs at this level. For certain overly emphasized high school programs in the United States this statement rings true as well. Also, we have recently seen the development of this semiprofessional mentality at some universities in Canada (notably in the West and the East).

It is true that today's highly competitive sport demands long, hard practice to reach the level of perfection necessary for winning records. So we must continually ask ourselves how far we should let this trend go--this pursuit of excellence. This question is especially pertinent in educational circles where boys and girls, and young men and women, are there to get an education and need so many other valuable experiences as well (such as learning to read, write, and cipher!).

Let me say quickly that I have no quarrel with a young person striving for excellence in competitive sport on a semiprofessional or professional basis. Why should anyone? After all, sport is a legitimate aspect of our culture. What I do get upset about, however, is what we permit to happen to a lot of boys and young men in Canadian hockey, for example, or what has happened to a very large extent with young men (and now young women too) in much of U.S. university sport--and so often with underprivileged youngsters too.

The Concept of the 'Semiprofessional'

It would help further if much of the sham and hypocrisy could be removed from competitive sport in both the United States and Canada. In other fields, the field of music, for example, the problem of amateurism, semi-professionalism, and professionalism has been resolved quite nicely. The person who plays the trumpet in the high school band is an amateur. If he or she is good enough to play with some group regularly on weekends for fifty dollars a night, then we can agree that semi-professionalism has been achieved. Who would be critical of this? Finally, this person might eventually choose to become a professional musician or music teacher as a lifetime occupation. At this point the individual really is a professional because his or her entire living will come from this source.

Such a graduated scheme has been viewed for a long time as quite acceptable in our society for musicians, artists, sculptors, actors, and many others--but somehow not for athletes! Why are athletes so different when it comes to involvement either within educational circles or on national- and international-level teams? Granted there have been breakthroughs in isolated instances (e.g., trust funds for downhill skiers, Olympic swimmers), but this has been accompanied by a lot of smirking and/or grimacing by die-hard purists.

A young athlete who takes money, or something else of intrinsic worth, may find that he or she is barred from so-called amateur athletics (although now some "dirty pro's" regularly achieve "pure" amateur status again because there is no semiprofessional category). There are still a great many people who believe that men and women athletes should not be permitted to accept any monetary return to support their efforts--but they wouldn't think of insisting upon this for young people in other areas of cultural endeavor. (Horrors! I am suggesting that sport is indeed an area of cultural endeavor!)

How Sport Became Singled Out

How did all of this come about historically--that is, the idea that an amateur athlete who took anything other than a varsity letter sweater for playing a favorite sport was a professional? Somehow in our background, some of the snobbish elitists in the late 1800s didn't want the "butcher boy from the other side of the tracks" imported to make a stronger team for the annual sporting competition of some upper-class group of sportsmen. This attitude soon resulted in a hoary tradition in Olympic competition. However, it is now obvious that what were leaks in the floodgates have rapidly developed into a deluge wherein millionaire basketball players and tennis stars grab much of the media attention at the Olympic Games.

Even well-intentioned members of state and provincial athletic associations tend to go overboard on this subject. However, we have finally outgrown the castigations and imposition of penalties that used to be meted out to university varsity swimmers who got paid during the summer for coaching younger swimmers at country clubs or municipal pools. Further, the idea that a college baseball player typically had to be careful as to which league he played in over the summer holidays has vanished. Finally, the ghost of Jim Thorpe is able to rest because Jim's withdrawn Olympic medals have now been returned to the bosom of the Thorpe clan (you remember those gold medals that were stripped from Jim because he accepted money for playing summer baseball).

Let's Make "Semiprofessional" Official

One answer to this longstanding impasse would be the official creation of a category designated as the semiprofessional. To be a bit facetious, I suppose we could argue that the National Collegiate Athletic Association in the States did just that a number of years ago. Only they called it the scholar-athlete, and with certain carefully defined--but often broken--stipulations they allow such a person to receive an athletic tender or scholarship.

Of course, they can now take it away at the end of a semester (for example) if the athlete "looks cross-eyed" at the coach or is injured. And now--woe unto us!--Canadian Inter-university Sport has permitted the introduction of limited athletic scholarships. However, they think that they can learn from the mistakes of the States and do it right--ha! ha!

Technically, if the officials enforced the spirit of the Olympic oath that the athletes all take, a great many young men and women would be barred from participating. I suppose the same thing could be said for our carded athletes in Canada. Now, however, even professional hockey players are "released" so that they can now play in Olympic competition, and the NHL may even interrupt its schedule for the next Winter Games. ("Avery Brundage, please stop spinning so rapidly in your grave!") However, the various Olympic officials have come to understand that they would be "torn from limb to limb" if they didn't look the other way. Then to save face, they and their international colleagues gradually altered the outmoded rules and regulations to conform to prevailing practice.

It's all part of the sham and hypocrisy that has built up around highly competitive sport--a most sordid mess to put it bluntly. Is it any wonder that our young people think us hypocrites when this topic arises, take their expenses and other "goodies" over and under the table, and then rush off offering their wares to the highest bidder as the next occasion arises?

One of the biggest laughs of all was when Canadian professional hockey all-stars blithely played the former U.S.S.R. "amateurs" for the world championship--and lost as often as not. In the meantime the semiprofessional Olympic hockey teams of both the United States and Canada took on these same "amateurs" in the Winter Olympics--and then headed for the nearest exit to sign as many professional contracts as might be available the minute the Olympic Games had been concluded. (But, never fear, that will soon all be "straightened out" when the pros will take over completely!)

I am not criticizing the young people here. They are simply "playing the game" that has been created by their elders, hypocrites who originally seemed so unwilling to adjust with the times. And now these officials "have thrown out the baby with the bath water!". Here I am referring to those men who have control of international sporting competition, and who quite willingly also accept the many perquisites that go along with this lifetime involvement.

Highly competitive sport today demands long, hard practice over a period of years. Most of our athletes simply could not afford to participate if they didn't receive more or less financial help. If highly competitive sport is worthwhile--and I realize this is a moot point under the commercialization and drug-oriented conditions that prevail all too often today--then we must give every boy and girl equal opportunity to take part regardless of family background. If this person (1) has the talent and (2) is truly prepared to sacrifice to become a great athlete, we should not hesitate to help him or her to the best of our ability to do so.

There Is One Major Caution

Further, if this deserving individual can be helped to work his or her way through college or university--even by virtue of athletic proficiency during the long summer break--we should still make this opportunity available. However, we must control overemphasis during the time when the athlete is officially registered in a university and taking a full schedule of bona fide classes. No other approach should be acceptable in Canada or anywhere else! The individual must be a registered student progressing normally toward a degree--even if it takes a bit longer. This is where Canada should continue to "part company" with the institutions that commercialize university sport in the United States. There is no other acceptable way.

Sport As a Socially Useful Servant

Finally, then, I have argued here that competitive athletics can hold great personal value for young men and women. Through their efforts these young people can make a significant social contribution as well. If we can't continue to work out ways that highly competitive sport and athletics will be a socially useful servant for the United States, for Canada, for the world, we should cut back sharply and tell the pros to go their own way. We have made mistakes in the past, and we are still making them. However, we still have it within our power to keep educational athletics in its proper perspective--in Canada and Division 3 intercollegiate athletics in the U.S. Let's make certain we distinguish carefully among the amateur, the semiprofessional, and the professional. Then let's insure that such criteria are scrupulously upheld. Only in this way we can hope that competitive sport will continue to serve the purposes for which it is intended.

PART III: HOW DO WE CORRECT THE SITUATION?

Chapter 13
How Sport Could Provide Experiences
Basic to World Peace

The world situation has become so threatening on a continuing basis that *all* professions should now work assiduously to make a contribution toward the goal of world peace. Keeping in mind that bona fide professions have historically developed codes of ethics which included an obligation to work for both the public good and that of the profession, this clearly means that the profession of physical education and educational sport has an obligation to foster and maintain societal values. There is an accompanying duty and responsibility on this continent for us to preserve and enhance the role of the sport and physical education profession as represented by the National Association for Sport and Physical Education in the United States (part of the AAHPERD), for example, and PHE Canada.

We believe that this profession has been highly traditional and has typically reacted to prevailing social conditions and pressures while rarely anticipating desired change in the culture. However, the world situation in relation to strategic nuclear power and other means of conducting warfare is such that the public good demands that we as the established sport and physical education profession join the fray in the struggle required to achieve lasting peace and international good will.

The late Laura J. Huelster (1982, p. 1) pointed out that,

. . . the survival of our society is threatened unless there is fitness to live the quality of life that de-emphasizes war and promotes peaceful solutions to national and international social, economic, and political conflicts. . . .

She argued further that general education should include knowledge about the conditions of human societies that are conducive to minimizing wars and maximizing peace. Huelster stressed additionally that a willingness to accept and act upon that knowledge depends not only upon convincing evidence, but also upon having attitudes and ideologies that are compatible with it.

What should be included in general education should undoubtedly be reflected in professional education as well. This is apparent because the highly threatening world situation makes us aware of the urgent need for a practical response so that future generations will possess both the knowledge and the accompanying attitudes to bring about a peaceful, productive state in the world.

Recommendations for Physical Activity Education (Including Educational Sport)

How can a field often known now as sport and physical education join in with any trend leading to such a future state? Keeping in mind (1) that its program should be directed to developmental physical activity in sport, exercise, and related expressive activities for people of all ages and conditions, and (2) that there is an urgent need to elevate compassionate-cooperative behavior to a level never deemed necessary before while discouraging and downplaying excessive violence, intimidation, unsportsmanlike conduct, and ignoring the spirit of the rules, what specific recommendations can be made at this time? Building on (and adapting) the tentative "principles," recommended by Huelster (1982, p. 19), the following recommendations are offered for serious consideration:

1. We should stress continually the cooperative elements and the need for more cooperative play in competitive games and sports.

2. We should reward through a variety of forms of recognition those who epitomize the qualities of fair play and sportsmanship that we wish to encourage.

3. We should make every effort to cope with overly aggressive competitive behaviors by redirecting them into more responsible cooperative ones. (In this regard, the profession should be exerting direct pressure on rules-making bodies to make sincere efforts to eliminate undue violence and aggression from their sports.)

4. We should insert the concept of 'individual freedom' to a much greater extent in sport and physical education programs by encouraging students to select freely the motor skills and play

forms they want to learn. (Understand that this recommendation does not apply to the student who seemingly doesn't want to be involved and possibly thereby improve his/her quality of life by developing such knowledge and competency.)

5. We should broaden program offerings to include more basic and exploratory motor skills such as (a) exercise patterns for physiological and/or psychological benefits, (b) body mechanics and relaxation techniques, (c) swimming and water safety knowledge and techniques, (d) lifetime individual and dual sports, (e) risk sports, and (f) expressive movement activities including folk, social, and modern dance.

6. We should, while developing such program offerings as in #5 above, use teaching and coaching strategies involving task-setting and problem-solving whenever appropriate. In the process, we should help students and clients to set performance-attainment goals beyond their expectations so as to promote the development of self-confidence.

Concluding Statement

Many social forces have become persistent historical problems that impact upon society and education directly (Zeigler, 1988, pp. 255-292). These problems are identified as (1) the influence of values and norms, (2) the type of political state, (3) the influence of nationalism, (4) the influence of economics, (5) the impact of organized religion, and (6) the need for ecological awareness. Two additional social forces have now been added to the list of persistent problems: (7) the impact of science and technology, and (8) the need for a search for world peace (Zeigler, 2002, p. 52)..

It will be difficult to convince the physical education and educational sport field to follow enthusiastically the recommendations made here. It will be especially difficult to persuade the many sport coaches who do not identify primarily with the organized sport and physical education educational field. Nevertheless, the goal of improved international understanding and eventual world peace is so vital, so all-compassing as we think of present trends and what may happen in this twenty-first century, that we should all think this subject through for with great care. We cannot simply leave it to "the other fellow" to do this for us.

Chapter 14
How Should We Judge Success
in Educational Sport Competition?

At the beginning of the 21st century, what does it mean when we speak about success in competitive sport or athletics? Does it mean that such-and-such a team won the championship of its league or conference? Or does success mean that you or your team won more games than you lost? Or does it possibly mean that you improved over your record of last year, and that your play this season was "respectable?" *Or does it only mean that today "I (or we) won, and you lost?"* ("We're Number 1!") These are some of the ways that most people would react if this question were asked of them. Which, if any, is the way that things ought to be--the way we would like them to be if we or our children and young people were playing on a team?

How can these questions be answered best? They are being answered one way by so-called major universities and colleges in the United States (NCAA Division I and IA, etc.) Their influence has unfortunately spread to other institutions and much of high school athletics as well. And, now more unfortunately, girls and women in the States, are also being caught in a "Catch 22" situation as they fight for equal status with men's overemphasized sport.

The Dilemma Facing Those Who Manage
Competitive Sport

This is the dilemma facing those who manage and coach competitive sport for both sexes every season in the "Excited" States. This is true whether it's conducted by a middle school, high school, college, university, or public or private agency. Consequently, because of undue pressure from the various media, this insidious influence is creeping into Canada steadily as well. The sponsors of these events demand a better answer than simply "Oh, this was a year for building character," and then laughing apologetically about such a weak response. (Interestingly, if team members really did "build character," they really should be bragging about it!)

In an eight-team basketball league, for example, only one team can win the championship title in a given year. What then can we say about the other seven teams--those that finished from second to eighth place? Are these teams and their members "losers" and whatever common epithets are typically used. Are the players on the teams that finished second to eighth basically inadequate human beings? Does a third-place finish in a gate receipt sport at the university level, for example, reflect so unfavorably on the organization that the coach should get fired from, or transferred elsewhere within, that educational institution? *With the almost disproportionate growth of sport as a social institution in society, these are questions that we simply must be ready to answer now and in the future.* The facile, but often sheepish and inadequate, responses offered at present, leave much to be desired.

It is obvious that the achievement of success in competitive sport is a complex matter. Help in answering the question as to what constitutes success can be obtained, for example, from a study by Professors Danylchuk and Chelladurai of The University of Western Ontario in which they researched the operative goals of intercollegiate athletics by testing the perceptions of athletic administrators in Canada. (Keep in mind that gate receipts are not an important factor in this conference.)

The athletic directors were asked to rank nine objectives (or operative goals) as follows: (1) entertainment, (2) national sport development, (3) financial, (4) transmission of culture, (5) career opportunities, (6) public relations, (7) athlete's personal growth, (8) prestige, (9) achieved excellence. The results were relatively homogeneous in ranking (1) transmission of culture, (2) athlete's personal growth, (3) public relations, and (4) prestige as the most important goals. Those athletic directors who were involved more heavily with athletic scholarships and recruitment gave higher ratings than the others to public relations, prestige, entertainment, and financial objectives.

What does all of this mean? Simply put, it means that *the determination of what constitutes "athletic success" is indeed a highly complex matter.* The media give major space, of course, to professional sport and semiprofessional university sport (especially in the States). Administrators in colleges and universities where commercialism is under control must counter at every turn the efforts of uninformed people to relate success only to an individual's or a team's won-loss record, or to the amount of money taken in at the gate. Athletic success can and should have a relatively different meaning for those who make up the institution's (or the agency's) internal and external environment.

What, then, should be considered sport or athletic success? School, college, university, recreation, and private agency administrators have too often been forced to consider the *extrinsic* results from sport competition. Now they also need desperately some yardsticks to help them assess the *intrinsic* worth of the various aspects of their competitive sport programs. These aspects or characteristics can indeed be evaluated. My recommendations regarding the more intrinsic characteristics of athletic success are as follows:

A high school, college, university, or public or private agency may claim athletic success *if and only if* the following occurs regularly at the following levels within your program:

The Individual

You have *athletic success* if the major objective in your program is with whether the person's growth, maturity, skill, and fitness are improved as a result of the athletic experience.

The Team

You have *athletic success* if an important objective in your program is with the quality of the competitive/cooperative experience, and whether there was sound improvement in the team's performance with a spirit of camaraderie and sportsmanship prevailing.

The Athletics Administrator

You have *athletic success* if the recognized concern of the sport/athletic administrator of your institution or agency is interpreting and carrying forward the philosophy and established policies and procedures of the institution or agency so that an efficient and effective program of competitive sport results.

The Coach (**and assistants**)

You have *athletic success* if your concern as a coach in your program is to be a dedicated professional educator who possesses great respect for the worth of the individual; who has an excellent knowledge and background in the sport in question; and who has the type of personality to inspire young men and women to achieve their potential within the demands of an educational environment.

The Game Officials

You have *athletic success* if your concern in your work is to provide qualified game and contest officiating that is carried out by officials who have an understanding and appreciation of the educational institutions or agencies in the league or conference in which they are officiating. (This may be difficult to evaluate.)

The Educational Institution or Agency

You have *athletic success* if the concern for your program is that the president, vice-presidents, deans, professors, and students (or the officers and executive of a public or private agency) have a true understanding of the educational and non-commercial objectives of the institution's or agency's athletics program for boys and girls and men and women and base their judgment of athletic performance accordingly.

The Board of Trustees, Education, or Governors

You have *athletic success* if the concern in your program is that the administrators make every effort to educate you and other board members so that you will evaluate athletic performance fairly, and so that you will understand the strengths and weaknesses of the program in keeping with the institution's or agency's avowed educational philosophy and its ability to support that position.

The Local Community

You have athletic success if the concern in your program is to work as constructively as possible with the media so that members of the local community are fully informed as to the institution's competitive sport philosophy and can share in the best

The State or Provincial Legislature

You have *athletic success* if the concern of your provincially supported or state-supported institution (or publicly or privately supported agency) is to make every effort to ensure that the elected members of the legislature understand the institution's or agency's competitive sport policy; that they have an opportunity for input into this policy's growth, development, and realization; and that they be fully aware of the dangers of excess commercialism as it affects such a valuable medium for the achievement of a sound educational/recreational experience for our young people. (This provision may have to be approached more indirectly in Canada than the United States because of different political structures.)

The Nation

You have *athletic success* if the concern in your program is to maintain the sport teams at all levels within the nation within an educational/recreational perspective so that citizens, including former participants and other supporters, may take pride in the overall achievement of the country's competitive sport program, *while at the same time keeping well in mind the fact that regular, often excessive media publicity may well mean that undesirable influences are present and should possibly be curtailed.*

The United States started going astray slowly but surely shortly after the turn of the twentieth century with its intercollegiate and inter-university sport. Despite all of the efforts of the rules-governing bodies, this trend has increased to the point where by and large the gate-receipt element has continued as a highly important factor in the intercollegiate sport picture. Additionally, varying percentages up to 90 % of Blacks, for example, in gate-receipt sports are not completing their degree programs in four years at these colleges and universities. Further, the effect of this unhealthy, commercialized development on high school sport has become most obvious as well.

Some may say that the 10 *characteristics* of athletic success presented above could be stated by the representatives of just about any school, college, or university, that their officials and coaches might think they are approximating the ideal now. However, these educational institution in the United States especially are often not living up to the letter of the inadequate rules. Further, the spirit of those statements hasn't a prayer of prevailing at present.

What Does This Mean Ultimately?

What does this means ultimately? It tells us that something at the core of the value structure is rotten and must somehow be rooted out. This is why improved evaluative techniques need to be developed, enforced, and maintained by national sports-governing bodies. And, to prevent ever-present undue pressures by alumni and businesspeople, the federal government itself should get involved to overcome such educational deficiency.

Some will argue that commercialism and excessive media attention do not necessarily mean that a program can't be educationally sound. This could conceivably be true, but much of the experience in the United States has shown that such a beneficial outcome is highly unlikely. It has now become a debatable question whether--under the prevailing conditions--sport does more harm than good.

Sadly, I have come to believe that only a naive person would think that Canada and other countries aren't falling prey to many of the same influences that have made helpless laughing stocks of many dignified, beleaguered, well-intentioned, yet overwhelmed university and college presidents in the United States. These administrators tried to take control, but they have consistently been shunted aside. If they as individual presidents become too obstreperous, they are forced to the sidelines. "The tail is wagging the dog in the States, and Canadians must struggle to keep their dog on an even keel on all four legs--and with a clear head too!"

Chapter 15
Why Don't We Have Sport *Critics*?

A "Professional Suicide" Note

In a 2000 issue of *Sport Illustrated*, Jeff MacGregor wrote what might be called a "professional suicide note" in his "Twilight of the Scribes" column. He opined that "sportswriters will soon be dinosaurs, driven to extinction by the Ice Age of the Internet." His thoughts are insightful if we duly consider the rapid advances being made in the Web-wired world.

His argument is interesting, but the demise of the sportswriter might be prophesied for a much better reason. The over-commercialism of competitive sport, with all of its attendant vices and vicissitudes, is gradually requiring an affiliated "element" much more basic than sports reporting or sports writing. *The time is overly ripe for the dawn of the sport critic!*

We Still Do Read Newspapers!

I believe also that MacGregor is jumping the gun with his debatable assertion that we don't presently depend on the printed word for our primary coverage of any one day's happenings. Watching news programs on TV, or listening to newscasts on the radio are helpful and timely, but they will never give an intelligent, informed citizen both the overall and the specific coverage that the daily newspaper provides. Moreover, when I carry my coffee cup into my den in the morning after breakfast, I have the local newspaper in my other hand.

A Desperate (Unrealized) Need for Sport Critics

The sports world, all of North American society for that matter, needs sports critics desperately. We need qualified professionals who day by day analyze and then assess critically what is truly happening in competitive sport. (Here I must insert, as two most rare examples of people who do [or did] this admirably, the names of Robert Lipsyte of *The New York Times* and Jay Weiner of the *Minneapolis Star-Tribune*.) Give us the scores and "who did what?" of course, but over and above that explain to us in a variety of insightful ways how sport as a social institution is doing more bad (evil) than good in society (or vice versa).

Frankly, a good case can be made today for the position that evil is winning out over what some of us thought--"in another world at another time"--was the case with competitive sport. Because of what has become a "cancer" growing dangerously on a supposedly beneficial social institution, today's sportswriters should involve themselves almost fully with sport criticism. However, with almost no exception, sportswriters are just that--sports***writers!*** They are not critics of the enormous social institution that commercialized sport has become.

Professionals: Need to Be More Professional

By asking for the advent of a *true* sport critic, not the ever-present sportswriter or overly enthusiastic, talking head television or radio announcer, I am neither attacking nor defending competitive sport. My immediate goal is to urge these people--as media *professionals*--to become much more objective in determining the advantages and disadvantages if sport for life. I want to be assured that in-depth involvement in sport today results in what we may call a "redeeming social value.: At present I feel that such an assertion is high debatable.

A Social Institution That Needs to Be Challenged

That is the issue, the real problem today. Sport must be challenged because it has become a highly powerful social institution without a well-defined theory. Other social institutions have underlying social theories, admittedly often conflicting. We need a general theory for the institution of sport. Such a theory should have some sort of a hypothetical form--"IF you do THIS in a particular way, THEN you should be able to expect THAT will result. *All that we know now is that,*

(1) if you have the inherent talent,

(2) if you have a sufficient means of support to get by financially,

(3) if you get the best possible coaching,

(4) if you spend an inordinate amount of time perfecting your skills,

(5) if you can control yourself (psychologically) under trying circumstances, and

(6) if you are willing to experiment with one or more of a great number of possible performance-enhancing substances--*and don't get caught!*--you MAY get a shot a making it to the top in a competitive sport, and you are highly successful, you could become extremely rich in everyday terms.

Who Should Be the Guardian?

The guardians of the "functional satisfaction" of sport should be the sportsman or sportswoman and the spectators, of course. The sport historian, the sport sociologist, and the sport philosopher should analyze all types of sport, using their respective research methodology and related techniques, in a scholarly manner. Additionally, the guardian of the applied ethics of sport should be the sport critic serving as a member of a trusted profession.

With regard to sport's role in society today, we are all akin to the proverbial blind person attempting to describe an elephant using the sense of touch only (i.e., here a trunk, there a tusk, etc.). We humans do have sight. Yet right now we are all people trying to assemble a jigsaw puzzle before seeing the picture on the box! Sports critics, if true professionals, should be there every day helping humanity se the big picture of competitive sport at all levels. If this were the case. we might some day find that competitive sport is indeed a social institution *helping* humanity progress toward the uncertain future.

Chapter 16
How Can We Make Sport More Socially Acceptable?

Nero is said to have fiddled while Rome burned! But then we are not certain that he had all of his mental faculties. Here I submit that we too are "fiddling while many aspects of competitive sport are catching fire!"

What do I mean by this? I mean basically that the human values and ethical conduct displayed at all levels of competitive sport are becoming increasingly more questionable with each new season. This is even more true as we move from amateur to semiprofessional and finally to professional sport.

Sport and Values Promotion

Competitive sport has become extremely popular in North America, as well all over the world. It exerts an enormous influence on the people who are involved either actively or passively as spectators. The question, however, is whether competitive sport is fulfilling its potential in the promotion of values in North America? If yes, that's fine. If not, however, this becomes a key ethical dilemma for us all.

The influence of the values held by our citizens is extremely important to our future, to any social system for that matter. These values may be classified as social values, educational values, artistic values, sport values, etc. The societal values of the United States and Canada are actually quite similar. How could they be very different considering our geographical location? The problem, however, is whether those values that are conceived of as representative of the ideal general character are being achieved.

Basic Social Values

As reasonable people we can accept that people in this North American culture are in agreement with such societal values as (1) governance by law, (2) individual freedom, (3) protection from injury, (4) equality of opportunity, (5) privacy, and (6) promotion of individual welfare.

If you agree, this means that the leaders in our society have a responsibility to see to it that these *good* values--as opposed to *bad* values such as the opposite of those listed above--are promoted to the extent possible in all of our cultural activities.

Sport Values Should Be Consistent With Societal Values

This means that the values present in sport, for example, should be largely identical with those present in other activities within society. But are they? Does highly competitive sport today truly represent and promotes the best and finest societal values? This is not a simple question to answer, but it is obviously most important.

Examining this matter carefully, we may be surprised to learn that sport's contribution to human wellbeing is a highly complicated matter. On the one side, there are those who claim that sport contributes significantly to the development of what are regarded as the *socio-instrumental* values--that is, the values of teamwork, loyalty, self-sacrifice, aggressiveness, and perseverance consonant with prevailing corporate capitalism in democracy and in most other political systems as well. In the process of making this "contribution," however, we discover also that there is now concern that in the process of contributing to the "global ideal" of capitalism, democracy, and advancing technology, sport has developed an ideal that opposes the historical, fundamental *moral* values of honesty, fairness, good will, sportsmanship, and responsibility in the innumerable competitive experiences provided).

I have personally tried to answer this question by presenting what I feel are the key ethical dilemmas facing sport. In other words, what bad values are we permitting when we should be fostering their opposite--that is, good values?

As I see it, the following should be eliminated before we can feel that North American sport is a positive social force:

Undue Violence in Hockey

The situation in hockey is disgraceful even though the penalty for initiating a fight has recently been stiffened. If a player did on the street what is often done on the ice, that offending individual would go to jail. Fighting and excessive violence spoils the demonstration of the rightful skills of the sport.

The Danger Inherent in Boxing

Boxing should not be permitted as a competitive sport, because the objective of a fighter is to render his opponent senseless. A human head simply cannot stand the pounding day in and day out. Because the "veneer of civilization" is often thing, however, this is not to say that we shouldn't teach "the manly art of self defense" with adequate safety equipment. However, much safer amateur wrestling accomplishes this objective better and more safely.

Excessive Commercialism:

This is not a problem in Canada in educational sport at any level, but it is a serious problem in U.S. intercollegiate athletics at the higher levels. And commercialism has definitely threatened the future of the Olympic Games. Undue commercialism is also the bottom line in professional sport and actually occasions a number of the other problems present today.

Excessive Nationalism in Olympic Sport

We all want the United States and Canada to do well in international sporting competition, but such accomplishment should be consistent with our population and the values held by each country, respectively. It is fine to win a gold medal, but this shouldn't result in financial security for life and take away from the contribution of the large majority of participants. They should also stop playing the national anthem of the gold medal winner.

Overemphasis in Professional Sport

Of course, there will be overemphasis in professional sport. Achieving excellence is important to the careers of those involved. But semiprofessional and amateur sport should be kept in perspective; the young man or woman should be guided to achieve maturity and to develop competencies and skills for his or her life goals.

Use of Performance-Enhancing Drugs

There are now between 400 and 500 banned substances that in one way or another might enhance sport performance. This makes it extremely expensive and almost impossible to discover the possible presence of any one drug in an athlete's system. We simply must stress the value of *fair* play as the young athlete develops in his or her sport.

Injuries in Collision Sports

Sports such as football and hockey occasion many serious injuries, the effects of some which do not appear until later life. This makes it vital that equipment and rules are designed for maximum safety. It is also imperative that athletic trainers be well qualified, and that fine medical practitioners and specialists are readily available when injuries occur.

Misuse of Power by Coaches

By the very nature of competitive sport, a basic tcnct of North American culture--a person's individual freedom--may very easily be abused daily by overly zealous coaches who rule over their charges too authoritatively. Society should see to it that adequate channels of appeal are available to athletes who may be maltreated in this regard.

Failure of Sports-Governing Bodies to *Establish* Creeds and *Enforce* Codes of Ethics

Some very feeble efforts have been made along this line, but by and large there are no carefully developed codes of ethics either for athletes or for coaches. Unsportsmanlike conduct abounds--that is, the "good" foul, trash-talking to opponents, showboating after a touchdown or a good play, the "dirty" play or "hidden" foul. There should be disciplinary systems established within the associated professions to discipline players and/or coaches for major and minor infractions of established code of ethics. Unless one of society's laws is actually broken, at present no one disciplines ethical malpractice either by players or coaches.

Conclusion

All of this adds up to one big question: *Is competitive sport a socially useful influence in society? If the answer is yes, that's fine; let's make it even better. If not, and there is much open to question in this regard, it should be cleared up or abolished.*

Chapter 17
The Olympic Games:
A Question of Values

There's a vocal minority who believe the Olympic Games should be abolished. There's another minority, including the Games officials and the athletes, who obviously feel the enterprise is doing just fine. In addition, there's a larger minority undoubtedly solidly behind the commercial aspects of the undertaking. They have a good thing going; they liked the Games the way they are developing--the bigger, the better! Finally, there's the vast majority to whom the Olympics are either interesting, somewhat interesting, or a bore. This "vast majority," if the Games weren't "there!" every four years, would probably agree that the world would go on just the same, and some other social phenomenon would take up their leisure time.

Ancient "Olympism"

Olympism has its roots in the beliefs of the ancient Greeks, who encouraged people to develop their physical, moral, intellectual, cultural and artistic qualities harmoniously. This meant taking part in a blend of sport, art, educational and cultural activities. This philosophy was celebrated through the Olympic Games, a festival involving athletes, scholars and artists from many cultural fields.

The Goal of Modern Olympism

Frenchman Pierre de Coubertin, who in 1894 led the re-establishment of the Olympic Movement, is recognised as the father of modern Olympism. He modernized ancient Greek ideals and launched them again to the rest of the world through the staging of a modern Olympic Games in 1896. Today, the festival celebrates the ideals that remain at the heart of Olympism. By blending sport with culture and education, Olympism promotes a way of life based on:

> The balanced development of the body, will and mind
> The joy found in effort
> The educational value of being a good role model
> Respect for universal ethics including tolerance, generosity, unity, friendship, non-discrimination and respect for others.

All in all, the claim is that the goal of Olympism is to sport to promote the balanced development of people as an essential step in building a peaceful world society that places a high value on human dignity.

Pray tell me, therefore, where in the noble sentiments expressed above does it even intimate that a country ought to strive to "own the podium," that athletes are defending their country's honor, that they should feel shame if they did their best and didn't win a medal, or—say—that multi-millionaire National Basketball Association professionals ought to represent their country of origin at the Games!

What a travesty it has all become! Thank goodness that many fine athletes don't believe this tripe that has been visited upon us! However, the people do love a spectacle, and the 2000 Olympic Games held in Sydney, Australia, for example, were a spectacle from start to finish. Sydney, Australia evidently wanted worldwide recognition. Without doubt, Sydney got recognition! The world's outstanding athletes wanted the opportunity to demonstrate their excellence. From all reports they had such an occasion to their hearts' and abilities' content. The International Olympic Committee, along with their counterparts in each of the 200 participating nations, earnestly desired the show to go on; it went on with a bang!

Sydney spent an enormous amount of money and energy to finance and otherwise support this extravaganza and surrounding competition. The IOC and its affiliates remained solvent for another four years, while Sydney contemplated its involvement with this enormous event and its aftermath. "Problem, what problem?" most people in the public sector would assuredly ask if they were confronted with such a question.

The Problem

This analysis revolves around the criticisms of the "abolish the Games group." Sir William Rees-Mogg (1988, pp. 7-8), is one of the Olympic Movement's most vituperative opponents. He believes the problem is of enormous magnitude. In fact, he lists fifteen sub-problems in no particular order of importance except for the first criticism that sets the tone for the remainder: "The Olympic Games have become a grotesque jamboree of international hypocrisy. Whatever idealism they once had has been lost. The Games now stand for some of the things which are most rotten and corrupt in the modern world, for prestige, nationalism, publicity, prejudice, bureaucracy, and the exploitation of talent" (p. 7).

It would not be appropriate to enumerate here *in great detail* the remaining 14 problems and issues brought forward by Rees-Mogg. Simply put, however, he stated that "The Games have been taken over by a vulgar nationalism, in place of the spirit of internationalism for which they were revived" (p.7). He decried also that, in addition to promoting racial intolerance, "the objectives of many national Olympic programmes is the glorification and self-assertion of totalitarian state regimes," often "vile regimes guilty of many of the crimes which the Olympic Games are supposed to outlaw" (p. 7).

Rees-Mogg decried further "The administration of the Olympic Games [that] is politically influenced and morally bankrupt" (p. 7). Additionally, at this point, he asserted that "the international bureaucracies of several sports have become among the most odious of the world." In this respect he lashes out especially at tennis, chess, cricket, and track and field. Still further, he charges that threats by countries to boycott the Olympics have time and again made it a political arena akin to the United Nations.

The messenger has not yet completed his message. Rees-Mogg condemns "the worship of professionally abnormal muscular development," and states that it is "a form of idolatry to which ordinary life is often sacrificed" (p. 7). Since these words were written in 1988, these problems have assuredly not been corrected. They have actually worsened (e.g., ever-more drugs to enhance performance, bribery of officials assigned to site selection). The entire problem of drug ingestion to promote bodily development for enhanced performance has now become legendary. Couple this with over-training begun at early ages in selected sports for both boys and girls, and it can be argued safely that *natural*, all-round development has been thwarted for a great many young people, not to mention the fact that only a minute number makes it through to "Olympic glory." More could be said, but the point has been made. Basically, Rees-Mogg has claimed that it has become a world "in which good *values* are taken by dishonest men and put to shameful uses" (p. 8).

Social Forces as Value Determinants

In the present discussion about the Olympic Games, it may be worthwhile to first take a brief look at the "Olympic Games Problem" from the standpoint of the discipline of sociology. This is because in an analysis such as this, the investigator soon realizes the importance of the major social forces (e.g., values, economics, religion) as determinants of the direction a society may take at any given moment. Sociology can indeed help with the question of *values*. For example, Parsons' complex theory of social action can be used to place any theory of social or individual values in perspective. His general action system is composed of four major analytically separable subsystems: (1) *the cultural system*, (2) *the social system*, (3) *the psychological system*, and (4) *the system of the behavioral organism.* The theory explains how these subsystems compose *a hierarchy of societal control and conditioning* (Johnson, 1969, pp. 46-58; Johnson, 1994, pp. 57 et ff.).

The cultural system at the top in the action-theory hierarchy provides the basic structure and its components, in a sense, thereby, programming the complete action system. The social system is next in descending order; it has to be more or less harmoniously related to the *functional* problems of social systems. The same holds for the structure and functional problems of the third level, the psychological system (personality), and the fourth level, the system of the behavioral organism (i.e., the individuals involved). Further, the subsystem of culture exercises "control" over the social system, and so on up and down the scale. Legitimization is provided to the level below or "pressure to conform" if there is inconsistency. Thus, there is a "strain toward consistency" among the system levels, led and controlled from above downwards.

What is immediately important to keep in mind is that there are *four levels of structure within the social system* itself (e.g., Hong Kong as a social system within Southeast Asia and, more recently, in its developing relationship with Mainland China's culture). Proceeding from the highest to the lowest level– i.e., from the general to the more specific–we again find four levels that are designated as (1) values, (2) norms, (3) the structure of collectivities, and (4) the structure of roles. All of these levels are normative in that the social structure is composed of sanctioned cultural limits within which certain types of behavior are mandatory or acceptable. Keeping in mind for the present discussion that *values are at the top* --the highest level--and that there are many categories of values (scientific, artistic, *sporting* , and values for personalities, etc.). These social values–including *sport* values too, of course–are simply assessments of the ideal general character for the social system in question. Finally, the basic point to keep in mind here is that *individual* values about sport will *inevitably* be "conditioned" by the social values prevailing in any given culture. In other words, there will be very strong pressure to conform.

Use of the Term "Value" in Philosophy

Moving from the discipline of sociology to that of philosophy, the investigator will use the term "value" as equivalent to the concepts of "worth" and "goodness." The opposite of these terms (i.e., "evil") will be referred to as "disvalue." It is possible, also, to draw a distinction between two kinds of value; namely, *intrinsic* value and *extrinsic* value. When a human experience has intrinsic value, therefore, it is good or valuable in itself--i.e., an end in itself. An experience that has extrinsic value is one that brings about goodness or value also, but such goodness or value serves *as a means to the achievement of something or some gain in life.*.

One of the four major subdivisions of philosophy has been called *axiology* (or the study of values). Until philosophy's so-called "Age of Analysis" became so strongly entrenched in the Western world at least, it was argued typically that the study of values was *the* end result of philosophizing as a process. It was argued that a person should develop a system of values consistent with his/her beliefs in the subdivisions of *metaphysics* (questions about reality), *epistemology* (acquisition of knowledge), and *logic* (exact relating of ideas). Some believed that values existed only because of the interest of the "valuer" *(the interest theory)*. *The existence theory*, conversely, held that values exist independently in the universe, although they are important in a vacuum, so to speak. They could be considered as essence added to existence, so to speak. A pragmatist (e.g., an experimentalist) views value in a significantly different manner (*the experimentalist theory*). Here values that yield practical results that have "cash value" bring about the possibility of greater happiness through more effective values in the future. One further theory, *the part-whole theory*, is explained by the idea that effective relating of parts to the whole brings about the highest values (Zeigler, 2010, p, 67).

Domains of Value Under Axiology

The study of ethics under axiology considers morality, conduct, good and evil, and ultimate objectives in life. There are a number of approaches to the problem of whether life, as humans know it, is worthwhile. Some people are eternally hopeful (*optimism*), while others wonder whether life is worth the struggle (*pessimism*). In between these two extremes there is the golden mean (*meliorism*) that would have humans facing life boldly while striving constantly to improve one's situation. In the latter instance it is not possible to make final decisions about whether good or evil will prevail in the world.

A second most important question under ethics is what is most important in life for the individual. This is a fundamental question, of course, in this discussion about human values in relation to the Olympic Games. What is the ultimate end of a person's existence? Some would argue that pleasure is the highest good (*hedonism*). One position or approach under hedonism in modern history is known as *utilitarianism*.. Here society becomes the focus, not the individual. The basic idea is to promote the greatest happiness for the greatest number in the community. Another important way of looking at the *summum bonum* (or highest good) in life is called *perfectionism*. With such an approach the individual is aiming for complete self-realization, and a similar goal is envisioned for society as well.

A logical progression following from an individual's decision about the greatest good in life is the standard of conduct that he or she sets for the "practice of living." A *naturalistic* approach would not have a person do anything that leads to self-destruction; self-preservation is basic. In the late 18th century in Germany, Immanuel Kant, known as an *idealist*, felt that a person should act on only what should be considered a universal law. Similarly, orthodox religion decrees that humans must obey God's wishes that have been decreed with a purpose for all humankind. *Pragmatism*, defined loosely, suggest a trial run in a person's imagination to discover the possible consequences of planned actions.

Continuing with this line of philosophic thought a bit further because of the obvious relationship it has to involvement with the Olympic Games in one way or another (i.e., as participant, official, coach, governing body member, advertiser, governmental official, what have you?), certain interests we develop are apt to guide people's conduct in life. Those who are too self-centered are egotistical (*egoism*), while those feel their life purpose is to serve others are called altruistic (*altruism*). Many would argue, however, that Aristotle's concept of the "golden mean" should be deemed best, a desirable aim for a person to fulfill with his or her life span.

There are, of course other areas of value under the axiology subdivision of philosophy over and above ethics that treats moral conduct (e.g., *aesthetics*, that has to do with the "feelings" aspects of a human's conscious life). Further, because there has been a need to define still further values in the life of humans, specialized philosophies of education and religion have developed, for example. This applies further to a a sub–department of the mother discipline of philosophy that has become known as sport philosophy. In sport philosophy, people would presumably make decisions about the kind, nature, and worth of values that are intrinsic to, say, the involvement of people in sport however defined.

An Assessment of the Problem

The problem, the author believes, is this: Opportunities for participation in all competitive sport–not just *Olympic* sport– moved historically from amateurism to semi-professionalism, and then on to open professionalism. The Olympic Movement, because of a variety of social pressures, followed suit in both ancient times and in the present. When the International Olympic Committee gave that final push to the pendulum and openly admitted professional athletes to play in the Games, they may have pleased most of the spectators and all of the advertising and media representatives. But in so doing the floodgates were opened completely, and the original ideals upon which the Games were reactivated were completely abandoned. This is what caused Sir Rees-Mogg to state that crass commercialism had won the day. This final abandonment of any semblance of what was the original Olympic ideal was the "straw that broke the camel's back." This ultimate decision regarding eligibility for participation has indeed been devastating to those people who earnestly believe that money and sport are like oil and water; they simply do not mix! Their response has been to abandon any further interest in, or support for, the entire Olympic Movement.

The question must, therefore be asked: "What should rampant professionalism in competitive sport at the Olympic Games mean to any given country out of the 200+ nations involved?" This is not a simple question to answer responsibly. In this present brief statement, it should be made clear that the professed social values of a country *should* ultimately prevail–and they *will* prevail in the final analysis. However, this ultimate determination will not take place overnight. The *fundamental social values* of a social system will eventually have a strong influence on the *individual values* held by most citizens in that country, also. If a country is moving toward the most important twin values of equalitarianism and achievement, for example, what implications does that have for competitive sport in that political entity under consideration? The following are some questions that should be asked *before* a strong continuing commitment is made to sponsor such involvement through governmental and/or private funding:

1. Can it be shown that involvement in competitive sport at one or the other of the three levels (i.e., amateur, semiprofessional, professional) brings about desirable *social* values (i.e., more value than disvalue)?

2. Can it be shown that involvement in competitive sport at one or the other of the three levels (i.e., amateur, semiprofessional, or professional) brings about desirable *individual* values of both an *intrinsic* and *extrinsic* nature (i.e., creates more value than disvalue)?

3. If the answer to Questions #1 and #2 immediately are both affirmative (i.e., that involvement in competitive sport at any or all of the three levels postulated [i.e., *amateur, semiprofessional, and professional* sport] provides a sufficient amount of social and individual value to warrant such promotion),*can* sufficient funds be made available to support or permit this promotion at any or all of the three levels listed?

4. If funding to support participation in competitive sport at any or all of the three levels (amateur, semiprofessional, professional) is *not* available (or such participation is *not* deemed advisable), should priorities—as determined by the expressed will of the citizenry—be established about the importance of each level to the country based on careful analysis of the potential social *and* individual values that may accrue to the society and its citizens from such competitive sport participation at one or more levels?

Concluding Statement

In this analysis the investigator asks whether a country should be involved with, or continue involvement with, the ongoing Olympic Movement—as well as all competitive sport—unless the people in that country first answer some basic questions. These questions ask to what extent such involvement can be related to the social and individual values that the country holds as important for all of its citizens. Initially, study will be needed to determine whether sport competition at either or all of the three levels (i.e., amateur, semi-professional, and professional) does indeed provide positive social and individual value (i.e., more value than disvalue) in the country concerned. Then careful assessment--through the efforts of qualified social scientists and philosophers--should be made of the populace's opinions and basic beliefs about such involvement. If participation in competitive sport at each of the three levels can make this claim to being a social institution that provides positive value to the country, these efforts should be supported to the extent possible--including the sending of a team to future Olympic Games. If sufficient funding for the support of *all* three levels of participation is *not* available, from either governmental or private sources, the expressed will of the people should be established to determine what priorities will be invoked.

References

Johnson, H. M. (1969). The relevance of the theory of action to historians. *Social Science Quarterlty 21*(2), 46-58.

Johnson, H. M. (1994). Modern organizations in the Parsonsian theory of action. In A. Farazmond, *Modern organizations: Administrative theory in contemporary society*, pp. 57 et ff. Westport, CT: Praeger.

Rees-Mogg, W. (1988). The decline of the Olympics into physical and moral squalor. *Coaching Focus, 8 (1988)*, 7.

Zeigler, E. F. (2010). *Philosophy of Physical Activity Education (Including Educational Sport)*, p. 67. Victoria, BC: Trafford.

PART IV: LOOKING TO THE FUTURE

Chapter 18
Sport Management Must Show Social Concern As It Develops Tenable Theory

Today sport and all other social institutions (e.g., religion, politics, economics) are confronted with the need to demonstrate that they are worthwhile and responsible. Sport managers should truly understand what sport's status is, and how and why sport such standing occurred. Difficult decisions, often ethical in nature, will have to be made as the members of the sport management societies worldwide strive to continue the development of this profession/discipline. These professionals need to decide to what extent they wish to live up to the broad ideals of the programs being promoted by public, semipublic, or private agencies for all types of people of all ages. Those involved with professional preparation and scholarly endeavor urgently need a theory and a disciplinary model to place professional preparation for administrative or managerial leadership within the field on a gradually improving, sound academic basis. Practitioners need an online service that provides them with scholarly applied findings as they seek to serve in the behaviorally oriented environment of today's world.

An Epoch in Civilization Approaches Closure...

An epoch in civilization approaches closure when the basic convictions of the majority of the populace are challenged by a substantive minority. It can be argued that indeed the world is moving into a new epoch as the proponents of postmodernism have been affirming over recent decades. Within such a milieu there are indications that the sport management profession is going to have great difficulty crossing this chasm, this so-called, postmodern divide (Zeigler, 2003, p. 93).

Nevertheless, there is no question but that sport has become recognized as one of humankind's fundamental social institutions. However, I believe that there are now strong indications that sport's presumed overall recreational, educational, and entertainment role in the "adventure of civilization" is not being fulfilled adequately. Municipal recreation programs, private sport clubs, and school sport programs are "doing the best that they can" often with limited funding. At the same time the commercialized sport establishment gets almost all of the media attention and is prospering as never before. Thus, an intelligent, concerned citizen can reasonably ask, "What evidence do we have that sport as a social institution is really making a positive contribution to society?" I find myself forced to ask whether commercially organized sport is actually "talking a better game than it plays." Where or what is sport management's tenable theory? Recalling the well-known fairy tale. I find that I must declare--not that "the king doesn't have any clothes on"--but that "The king should prove (to society) that he is sufficiently clothed to justify our continuing support."

The sport industry is obviously "charging ahead" driven by capitalistic economic theory that overemphasizes ever-increasing gate receipts with an accompanying corollary of winning fueled somehow by related violence. One of the "principal principles" of physical education espoused in the early 1950s by Dr. Arthur Steinhaus (George Williams College) was that "sport was made for man, not man for sport"(1952). It is being countermanded day by day, week by week at all levels around the world. Interestingly, but disturbingly, a societal majority seems to lend support to this surge in the popularity of professionalized competitive sport. The athletes--those happy people on the way to the bank who do not mind being used as commodities--typically don't understand what is happening. They don't even recognize this as a problem. Neither do many (most?) aspiring sport management students in professional programs.

Sport Management Goes With the Tide

Everything considered, I am therefore forced to ask, "What are we helping to promote--we who have associated ourselves with sport management--and exactly why are we doing it?" I fear that we are simply going along with the seemingly inevitable tide. In the process we have become pawns to the prevailing sport establishment by "riding the wrong horse." Our present responsibility--to the extent that we are educators and scholars--should be to devote our efforts to provide sport management with tenable theory. This tenable theory should relate to sport and physical activity involvement for all people of all ages in society be they normal, accelerated, or special in status.

Governmental agencies sponsoring "amateur" sport competition should be able to state in their relationship to sport that: if "such-and-such" is done with reasonable efficiency and effectiveness through the sponsorship of sporting activities, then "such-and-such" will (in all probability) result. Personnel in these same agencies are striving to do just this, but not necessarily in an acceptable way consonant with overall societal values. Instead of working assiduously for a "from-the-ground-up" development of young athletes in the hope that they would achieve relatively superior status eventually, they are proceeding in what might be called a fast-track approach. By that I mean that governments are focusing primarily on the recruitment and development of potentially elite athletes who somehow come to their attention, athletes whom they hope will bring fame and glory to their country. So, again, I ask, where is the evidence that organized sport's goal is based on tenable theory consonant with societal values that claim to promote the welfare of all?

Need for a Broadened Outlook in Sport Management

I am heartened, however, by a number of recent publications in the *Journal of Sport Management* that discuss future directions in research. Frisby's EFZ Lecture (2005) , in referring to "The Good, The Bad, and The Ugly" strikes just the right note in her conclusion by urging a broadened outlook for sport management. Next Costa's study (2005) using Delphi technique provided excellent discussion based on the opinions of leaders in the field as to future directions. Concern was expressed about the ability to achieve the goals outlined (e.g., additional cross-discipline research) within our own discipline. Then, the entire "Expanding Horizons" issue offered interesting insights and approaches about research for consideration (2005). Finally, Chalip's analysis in his 2005 EFZ Lecture titled "Toward a distinctive sport management discipline," points us toward the achievement of "distinctive relevance" for our field. (This idea of a distinctive approach for a sport-management model strikes a resounding chord with me. Below I will seek to add a bit to the profession's consideration of this problem.)

Fortunately, also, there is a growing minority within the populace that supports a more humanistic position that accepts the steadily mounting evidence that all people--not just elite athletes striving for personal fulfillment and fame--need to be active in physical recreational activities throughout their entire lives. This leads me to inquire as to what role the professional sport management societies worldwide should play in the guidance of its members toward this end. Hopefully these men and women, serving as qualified professionals seeking the achievement of their society's most desirable values, will increasingly be in a position to assist sport and related physical activity to serve all people in our world society in the best possible way.

Before such a dream can become a reality, however, we need to dig deeply in our respective "cultural psyches" to begin to understand how society got itself in the presently questionable situation. Until at least the majority of people in our world's culture understand what has happened, what should be done, and what can be done, there is little hope for improvement in what I believe to be an increasingly untenable situation.

The Enlightenment Ideal Has Been Overturned

In retrospect, the 18th century in the Western world witnessed revolutionary thought that had caused it now to be known as the Age of Reason (or "enlightenment"). This outlook was based on ideals of truth, freedom, and reason for all humans. In the United States, however, the Enlightenment vision of Thomas Jefferson that promised political and social liberation was somehow "turned upside down." What happened in American life in the 19th century was that "progress" came to mean "technocratic progress." This was not the anticipated social progress for all people that was planned by the inculcation of such values as justice, freedom, and self-fulfillment. These vital goals of a democratic political system were simply subjugated to the more immediate instrumental values. As Leo Marx explains, this technological advancement "became the fulcrum of the dominant American world view" (p. 5).

In the realm of physical (activity) education there was a "battle of the systems" of exercise and gymnastics that took place in the final quarter of the 20th century. However, it was the burgeoning interest in sport that permitted sport to infiltrate in the program of school physical education as sport skills. This type of experience was expanded further in (what was termed) extracurricular activity with team sports for the more highly skilled boys and girls. Earlier physical education programs, where available, as well as programs in wartime eras, undoubtedly stressed the concept of education "of the physical" more than the "roll-out-the-ball" approach so evident in physical education in subsequent decades. There was also the concept of "education through the physical" was also promoted to a degree by the educational "progressivists" influenced by Deweyan pragmatism. Typically this broader emphasis waned during periods of war and international unrest.

Careful historical analysis of this situation has led me to believe that the steady development of the social institution of competitive sport in the United States over the past 150 years has reached a crossroads (Zeigler, 2005, Chaps. XI & XII). If a claim can reasonably be made that organized sports may be doing as much harm as it does good can be made, I am forced to ask, "Where is the sport management theory needed to refute such a proposition?" In the United States especially, and in much of the remainder of the world, there is seemingly little awareness that such a negative contention about organized sport can be made. The developing world permits without question the commercialization that has brought about sport's expansion and current gargantuan status. The conventional wisdom seems to be that "highly organized sport is good for people and our country. The more involvement an individual can have with sport, either actively or passively, the better he or she will be."

In the meantime, however, the vast majority of the population is getting inadequate involvement in regular, physical activity designed to help them live healthy, active, fulfilling lives. Many of these same people now possess--what Herbert Spencer in the mid-nineteenth century--called "seared physical consciences" He argued that in increasingly urbanized society there is inadequate physical activity education in the schools (1949). These same people simply don't know or appreciate what vigorous physical health "feels like." At the same time throughout their lives they are constantly being encouraged to pay increasing amounts of money to watch "skilled others" play games. (The resultant inactivity has created a crisis situation that will be discussed in some detail below.)

Hard Questions About Present Social Institutions

Social institutions are created and nurtured within a society ostensibly to further the positive development of the people living within that culture. Take democracy, for example, as a type of political institution that is currently being promoted vigorously by the United States throughout the entire world. (Such worldwide change will take time!) Within this form of social development, democracy has "struck up a deep relationship with economics and has found an eager bedfellow with whom to associate"--i.e., the institution of capitalism. Economics, of course, is another vital social institution upon which a society depends fundamentally. As world civilization developed, a great many of the world's countries have enacted with almost messianic zeal the promotion of such social institutions as democracy, capitalism, and --now!--an increasing involvement with competitive sport. The "theory" is that the addition of highly competitive sport to this mix will bring about more "good" than "bad" for the countries involved. But has it? Disturbing questions have now begun to arise in various quarters.

What does this all mean as we move along in the 21st century? Think of the example being set in North America, for example. Is there reasonable hope that the present brand of "combined" democratic capitalism that uses up the world's environmental resources inordinately will somehow improve the world situation in the long run? Can we truly claim with any degree of certainty that this "mix" of democracy and capitalism (with its subsequent inclusion of big-time sport) is producing more "good" than "bad"? (Admittedly, we do need to delineate between "what's 'good'" and "what's 'bad'" more carefully) There is no escaping the fact that the gap economically between the rich and the poor is steadily increasing. This means that "the American dream for all" is beginning to look like a desert mirage. Will the historical "Enlightenment Ideal" remain as an unfulfilled dream forever?

One of the results of the increasing development of the social institution of competitive sport is the creation of sport management societies in the respective regions and countries where such expansion has occurred. At the same time the question may be asked whether this development has reached a point where a claim can be made that highly competitive sport as a social phenomenon may be doing more harm than good in society. It is not that competitive sport does not have the potential for good that is being questioned here. (The world seems to have accepted this as fact!) It's the way that it is being carried out that is the problem. The world community does not really know whether this contention is true or not. However, sport's expansion is permitted and encouraged almost without question in all quarters. "Sport is good for people, and more involvement with sport of almost any type--extreme sport, professional wrestling--is better" seems to be the conventional wisdom. Witness, also, the millions of dollars that are being parceled out of tax revenues for the several Olympic enterprises perennially. So long as it's thought that "a buck's to be made," also, permit even Evander Holyfield to box professionally in what's called a sport until he won't be able to remember his own name!

In the meantime, the large majority of the population in the developed world is getting inadequate involvement in physical activity, with obesity increasing unduly at all ages and levels. This is a highly significant problem that is increasing daily. Conversely there is rampant starvation in the underdeveloped world where most people, including children, must labor inordinately just to survive. At the same time the public in the technologically developed world is being expected to pay increasing amounts of money to watch "skilled others," either on television or "in the flesh," play types of games and sports increasing in complexity and danger almost exponentially. At the same time, "The National Institutes of Health estimates that Americans will take five years off the average life span," reports Randolph in "The Big, Fat American Kid Crisis" (*The New York Times*, 2006). The eventual outcome of what is happening today can be encapsulated in the grim predictions that the bulk of children and youth in the coming generation of the developed world may be the first to die before their parents because of obesity, less physical activity, and related health problems.

Resultantly, I am forced to ask "What really are we promoting, and do we know why are we doing it?" I do not have a complete answer to these questions, of course. But I do believe this strongly: we need to develop a theory of sport that will permit us to assess whether what we call "competitive sport" is fulfilling its presumed function of promoting good in a society. To achieve this. we will need to establish connections and relationships with a variety of disciplines in the academic world. Some that come to mind immediately are sport sociology, sport history, sport psychology, sport philosophy, sport economics, as well as selected other fields where research findings could well have application to sport and related physical activity. Some of these fields are anthropology, social geography, and political science--all academic fields that could well help in any assessment of the findings of sport management.

I want to emphasize, also, that the field of sport management must keep a healthy balance between the theoretical and the practical in its ongoing scholarship and research. To do otherwise would be courting the same fate that befell the former Philosophic Society for the Study of Sport (now the IAPS). I'm sad to report that sport philosophy "went disciplinary" in the late 1960s and has never descended from that lofty perch. As the third president, my warning on this point in 1975 was to no avail (Zeigler, 1976). Today the International Association for Sport Philosophy has very few members and "they speak to no one," relatively speaking, except each other. This is an outcome that the field sport management will need to guard against assiduously. (Nevertheless, the disciplinary aspects of sport management should be pursued diligently, but there must be an accompanying pragmatic emphasis on applied research that is regularly and consistently downloaded to the "real world" where sport in its many forms takes place daily.)

Sport should be conducted in its various settings now and in the future, both generally and specifically, in a manner that will encourage its proper professional, educational and recreational uses, as well as its semiprofessional and professional concerns To guarantee such a state of affairs, sport must be challenged on an ongoing basis by people at all levels in a variety of ways. If this were to be the case, sport might possibly regain and retain those aspects that can contribute significant value to individual and social living.

In making these assertions, I must first define my terms accurately so that you are fully aware of what I am seeking to explain and also critique here. This is necessary because the term "sport," based on both everyday usage and dictionary definition, still exhibits radical ambiguity. Such indecision undoubtedly adds to the present confusion. So, when the word "sport" is used here, it will refer--unless indicated otherwise--to "competitive physical activity, an individual or group competitive activity involving physical exertion or skill, governed by rules, and sometimes engaged in professionally" (*Encarta World English Dictionary*, 1999, p. 1730).

Analyzing Sport's Role in Society

In this process of critiquing competitive sport, I believe further that society should strive to keep sport's drawbacks and/or excesses in check to the greatest possible extent. In recent decades we have witnessed the rise of sport throughout the land to the status of a fundamentalist religion. For example, we find sport being called upon to serve as a redeemer of wayward youth, but--as it is occurring elsewhere--it is also becoming a destroyer of certain fundamental values of individual and social life.

Wilcox (1991), for example, in his empirical analysis, challenged "the widely held notion that sport can fulfill an important role in the development of national character." He stated that "the assumption that sport is conducive to the development of positive human values, or the 'building of character,' should be viewed more as a belief rather than as a fact." He concluded that his study did "provide some evidence to support a relationship between participation in sport and the ranking of human values" (pp. 3, 17, 18, respectively).

Assuming Wilcox's view has reasonable validity, those involved in any way in the institution of sport--if they all together may be considered a collectivity--should contribute a quantity of redeeming social value to our North American culture, not to mention the overall world culture (i.e., a quantity of good leading to improved societal well-being). On the basis of this argument, the following questions are postulated initially for possible subsequent response by concerned agencies and individuals (e.g., federal governments, state and provincial officials, philosophers in the discipline and related professions):

(1) Can, does, or should a great (i.e., leading) nation produce great sport?

(2) With the world being threatened environmentally in a variety of ways, should we now be considering an "ecology" of sport in which the beneficial and disadvantageous aspects of a particular sporting activity are studied through the endeavors of scholars in other disciplines as well?

(3) If it is indeed the case that the guardian of the "functional satisfaction" resulting from sport is (a) the sports person, (b) the spectator, (c) the businessperson who gains monetarily, (d) the sport manager, and, in some instances, (e) educational administrators and their respective governing boards, then who in society should be in a position to be the most knowledgeable about the immediate objectives and long range aims of sport and related physical activity?

(4) If the answer to question No.3 immediately above is that this person should be the trained sport

and physical activity management professor, is it too much of a leap to also expect that person's professional association (!) to work to achieve consensus about what sport and closely related physical activity should accomplish? Further, should the professional association have some responsibility as the guardian (or at least the assessor) of whether the aforementioned aims and objectives are being approximated to a greater or lesser degree?

Answering these questions is a truly complex matter. First, as I have stated above, sport and related physical activity have become an extremely powerful social force in society. Secondly, if we grant that sport now has significant power in all world cultures--a power indeed that appears to be growing--we should also recognize that any such social force affecting society can be dangerous if perverted (e.g., through an excess of nationalism or commercialism). With this in mind, I am arguing further that sport has somehow achieved such status as a powerful societal institution without an adequately defined underlying theory. Somehow, most of countries seem to be proceeding generally on a typically unstated assumption that "sport is a good thing for society to encourage, and more sport is even better!" And yet, as explained above, the term "sport" still exhibits radical ambiguity based on both everyday usage and dictionary definition. This obviously adds even more to the present problem and accompanying confusion.)

As we consider this matter more seriously, we may be surprised. We may well learn that sport is contributing significantly in the development of what are regarded as the *social* values--that is, the values of teamwork, loyalty, self-sacrifice, and perseverance consonant with prevailing corporate capitalism in democracy and in other political systems as well. Conversely, however, we may also discover that there is now a great deal of evidence that sport may be developing an ideal that opposes the fundamental moral virtues of honesty, fairness, and responsibility in the innumerable competitive experiences provided (Lumpkin, Stoll, and Beller, 1999).

Significant to this discussion are the results of investigations carried out by Hahm, Stoll, Beller, Rudd, and others in recent years. The Hahm-Beller Choice Inventory (HBVCI) has now been administered to athletes at different levels in a variety of venues. It demonstrates conclusively that athletes will not support what is considered "the moral ideal" in competition,

As Stoll and Beller (1998) see it, for example, an athlete with moral character demonstrates the moral character traits of honesty, fair play, respect, and responsibility whether an official is present to enforce the rules or not. Priest, Krause, and Beach (1999) reported, also, that--over a four-year period in a college athlete's career--ethical value choices showed decreases in "sportsmanship orientation" and an increase in "professional" attitudes associated with sport.

On the other hand, even though dictionaries define social character similarly, sport practitioners, including participants, coaches, parents, and officials, have come to believe that character is defined properly by such values as self-sacrifice, teamwork, loyalty, and perseverance. The common expression in competitive sport is: "He/she showed character"--meaning "He/she 'hung in there' to the bitter end!" [or whatever]. Rudd (1999) confirmed that coaches explained character as "work ethic and commitment." This coincides with what sport sociologists have found. Sage (1998. p. 614) stated that "Mottoes and slogans such as 'sports builds character' must be seen in the light of their ideological issues" In other words, competitive sport is structured by the nature of the society in which it occurs. This would appear to mean that over-commercialization, drug-taking, cheating, bribe-taking by officials, violence, etc. at all levels of sport are simply reflections of the culture in which we live. Where does that leave us today as we consider sport's presumed relationship with moral character development?

This discussion about whether sport's presumed educational and recreational roles have justification in fact could go on indefinitely. So many negative incidents have occurred that one hardly knows where to turn to avoid further negative examples. On the one hand we read the almost unbelievably high standards stated in the Code of Conduct developed by the Coaches Council of the National Association for Sport and Physical Education (2001). Conversely we learn that today athletes' concern for the presence of moral values in sport declines over the course of a university career (Priest, Krause, and Beach, 1999).

With this as a backdrop, we learn further that Americans, for example, are increasingly facing the cost and consequences of sedentary living (Booth & Chakravarthy, 2002). Additionally, Malina (2001) tells us that there is a need to track people's involvement in physical activity and sport across their life spans. Finally, Corbin and Pangrazi (2001) explain that we haven't yet been able to devise and accept a uniform definition of wellness for all people. The one thought that emerges from these various assessments is as follows: We give every evidence that we desire "sport spectaculars" for the few much more than we want people of all ages and all conditions to have meaningful sport and exercise involvement throughout their lives.

Sport Management Theory and Practice

Defined traditionally, we might say that the sport manager is one who plans, organizes, staffs, leads (or directs), and controls (i.e., monitors and evaluates) progress toward predetermined goals within programs of sport for people of all ages, be they in normal, accelerated, or special populations. To place the current topic in historical perspective (i.e., the beginning of investigation about the management [or administration] of sport and physical activity in educational institutions largely), master's and doctoral degrees about the subject within departments and schools of education in the United States were completed initially at Columbia Teachers College and New York University starting in the mid-1920s. Individually, there were many well-intended, seemingly worthwhile studies completed. However, it was impossible to say what these--literally--thousands of investigations "added up to" 35 years later at the beginning of the 1960s decade was really not known.

In the 1960s, however, research and scholarship in administrative theory and practice related to physical education and athletic administration began to receive attention in several quarters. Through the efforts of King McCristal (dean) and the author (University of Illinois, U-C), we were able to get this area included as one of six subject-matter areas in the Big Ten Body-of-Knowledge Project. In the fall of 1972, a symposium was held on the subject at The University of Michigan, Ann Arbor. In a volume published in 1975, the results of 20 doctoral dissertations carried out at Illinois were published (Zeigler and Spaeth, 1975). However, financial and other constraints in higher education of the 1970s slowed this development down considerably.

Then the rise of a so-called disciplinary approach to the field of physical education, plus the perennial claim of the "educational essentialist" that it is only the hard sciences that provide the basic knowledge, resulted in the introduction of the term kinesiology to supplement (or even supplant!)

that of physical education at the university level. This tended to severely downgrade the importance of administrative theory and practice programs within the field, while job opportunities for professors related to biomechanics, exercise physiology, and motor learning increased. Concurrently, however, burgeoning interest in commercialized, highly competitive sport within higher education and in the public sector created a need for the establishment and development of college and university curricula in sport management. So the essence of what was often being eliminated in one program appeared to be springing up in a new curriculum stream--sport management. It was at this point on February 24, 1986 that a small group of us witnessed the successful creation of the now-successful North American Society for Sport Management.

Most of those behind the establishment of NASSM actually envisioned an association with a broad emphasis leading to the promotion of sport and physical activity for all people of all ages. However, interest in highly organized, elite sport seems to have "engulfed" conference presentations in the various aspects of competitive sport management. Sport management has rapidly become a mushrooming field in its own right that increasingly has its own curriculum independent of former physical education and athletics administration courses in educational institutions. Concurrently, the "eager scientists" in kinesiology, who conceptually relegated administrative theory and practice for physical education and athletics to the dustbin insofar as its place in their disciplinary curriculum is concerned, are presumably now quite happy and relieved in those sites where such separation has actually occurred.

Intramural and recreational sport is actually doing quite well at the college and university level, but is almost nonexistent at the high-school level and lower. Finally, the near demise of physical activity programs "for the many"--required within education at all levels within education prior to 1950--does not even appear on the radar screen of the large majority of professional preparation personnel in universities. Yet, because of the decline of required physical education, it has become starkly apparent that the health and physical fitness of the populace needs a strong shot in the arm to again establish a firm foothold in public consciousness. (It doesn't seem that the "War on Terrorism" will bring this change. Do we need another world war to accomplish this?) This is true even though--almost daily--reports of scientific studies tell us of the beneficial effects of regular physical activity on the human organism in so many different ways.

In such a developing world environment, then, what is the mission of a field called sport management, still a fledgling profession but one that is rapidly catching on all over the world? Frankly, I believe strongly that our profession needs to understand (define?) its mission much better than appears to be the case at present. Exactly what is its fundamental purpose in society? Further, how does the mission of sport management globally relate to the mission of the various professional associations composed primarily of men and women involved in the professional education of future sport managers? (Keep in mind that the typical professional sport promoters worldwide presently live in "another world"!)

Unfortunately, as I see it, the outlooks or aims of those people who today promote sport competition professionally, and that of those who believe they are promoting such competition educationally, appear to be getting closer all the time. I am referring here to the people involved, for example, in the National Basketball Association or the National Collegiate Athletic Association in the United States, respectively. Granted that the people in both of these associations are operating on the assumption that the provision of highly competitive sport opportunities in society is a good thing. Also, they appear to believe that promoting ever more opportunity for the masses to observe such activity is worthwhile. The fact that the cultivation of a "fan club" for professional sport also provides exorbitant income for the "accelerated few" athletes and a dubious future for the vast majority of athletes who don't "make it" appears to be of little concern. This is unfortunate for that "vast majority" because their educational background has typically been stunted by excessive involvement in competitive sport while enrolled at universities.

Frankly, I believe this assumption of "goodness " for society has become a dubious premise or principle upon which most of these promoters and/or educational administrators are operating. I maintain that this is so unless they can provide accompanying evidence to substantiate to society that the continuation and enlargement of the present trend to increasing commercialization in sport is contributing positively to society as a social institution. To repeat, all social institutions must have an underlying theory to justify their continuing existence. The basic question, I submit. is simply this: In this evolving situation, what kind of "good"--philosophically speaking--can we claim is currently being made by competitive sport?

To one who has followed and written extensively about this development down through the 20th century from both a historical and a philosophical standpoint, I can only report (sadly!) that the excesses and corruption of competitive sport have increased steadily decade by decade. And, even more sadly, the seemingly jaded public (as fans) does not seem to realize--or seems to accept--that sport's status as a desirable social institution is being lowered steadily with each passing year. (I won't even get into the question of the taking of one or more of 400-500 drugs to enhance performance that the sport establishment is facing today.) Competitive sport is forced to stay within the law, but its typically laudable creed espoused so freely requires an enforceable code of ethics in the present--not as a dream for the future.

Concurrently, the low status perennially accorded to physical education-- except in times of war when referred to as "physical fitness"--continues. This is true even though ongoing research in kinesiology and physical education--and the field's related disciplines--is steadily making the case for regular, developmental physical activity as an essential, if not a vital, social institution to be employed for the benefit of all. Nevertheless the term "sport," and what it connotes to the average mind, largely overrides the need for the provision of necessary funding of developmental physical activity as a social institution. I firmly believe that provision for the managing and promoting developmental physical activity in sport, exercise, and physical recreation for people of all ages, be they part of accelerated, normal, or special populations, should at least be an auxiliary part of our mission in sport management. Yet we find that our professional associations and disciplinary societies relayed to "physical activity" are steadily and increasingly becoming more disjointed as they grow farther apart. Other professions and disciplines are "filling in" where we should be "producing" (e.g., recreation, medicine).

You can see where I am heading with this analysis. I believe it is now incumbent upon the field of sport management (i.e., these professional organizations worldwide) to investigate and subsequently understand precisely what effect sport, however defined and with all of its ramifications, is having on society. Is it more good than bad? Who knows? The professional and semiprofessional sport managers can't answer this basic question. (Many probably wouldn't want to know anyhow if it meant a possible shifting of emphasis in their offerings.) Therefore I urge the world's various professional sport management associations to take a hard look at what appears to be a steadily growing problem. They need to determine (1) what effect sport is having on society; (2) if there is a problem with the present development, and to what extent the professional associations (e.g., in North America) may unwittingly be part of the problem; and (3) in what ways professional sport management associations can ensure that sport as a whole, and more specifically its many programs at all levels, are moving in the right direction? These questions can't be answered satisfactorily without an underlying theory of sport management that meets the needs of all people.

Need for a Theory of Sport Management

Returning to the assertion made earlier, a theory underlying sport management could contribute greatly to the answering of the questions raised immediately above. It would need to be related basically to the social sciences and to certain professions that carry out their own independent research as well (e.g., business administration). It should contain "propositions of fact" that can, at least in principle, be verified empirically. "Propositions of value" are subjective and therefore typically conform to societal values and norms. Therefore, it would not be a philosophy of sport management, although a concerned individual or group might well philosophize about such human activity.

A theory is not a taxonomy, however, although a taxonomy of sport management will necessarily evolve as scientific and scholarly investigation about it is carried out. "A taxonomy may be defined as a classification of data according to their natural relationships, or the principles governing such classifications…In fact, one could probably make a good case to support the contention that any science begins with a taxonomy…" (Griffiths, 1959. p. 17)

A Taxonomy for Sport Management. Below as Table 1, I have included a sample of what a taxonomy of sport management might look like. It includes both scholarly and professional dimensions with three headings defined as (1) areas of scholarly study and research, (2) related disciplinary aspects, and (3) professional aspects. The possibility of "streaming" is mentioned at the undergraduate level. Also, there are three categories of graduate education postulated.

(Note: Reactions and/or recommendations for change or additions to Table 1 would be appreciated at <zeigrog@uniserve.com>)

Table 1

SPORT MANAGEMENT:
SCHOLARLY AND PROFESSIONAL DIMENSIONS

Areas of Scholarly Study & Research	Related Disciplinary Aspects	Professional Aspects
I. BACKGROUND, MEANING, & INTERCULTURAL SIGNIFICANCE	-History -Philosophy -International & Comparative Study	-International Relations -Professional Ethics
II. SOCIO-CULTURAL & BEHAVIORAL ASPECTS	-Sociology -Economics -Psychology (individ.& social) -Anthropology -Political Science -Geography -Law	-Application of Theory to Practice
III SPORT MANAGEMENT THEORY	-Management Science -Business Administration (e.g., sport marketing sport finance, facility management, sales)	-Application of Theory to Practice
IV. CURRICULUM THEORY & PROGRAM DEVELOPMENT	-Curriculum Studies	-Application of Theory to Practice

1. *General Education*: universities and colleges typically have a distribution requirement for all students in the humanities, social-science, and natural sciences.

2. *Professional* Core Subjects: an irreducible minimum requirement in the following subjects is required: communication & media relations, economic theory & sport finance, sport marketing, sponsorship & sales, legal aspects, sport governance, sport ethics, the international sport industry, and sport & physical activity internships.

3. *Specialized* Undergraduate Professional Preparation; streaming possibilities may be added in the degree program.

4. *Graduate* Education; three types of specialization are desirable: (1) professional preparation stream; (2) disciplinary stream, (3) practitioner stream)

V. MEASUREMENT & EVALUATION	-Theory about the Measurement Function	-Application of Measurement Theory of Practice

162

A Model for Sport Management: The development of a model, or taxonomy, could be important for evolving theory because it would enable a researcher not only to ask questions, but also to speculate as to how they might be answered. The term "model" has a number of meanings. The one that concerns a developing theory of sport management would be: "a description of a set of data in terms of a system of symbols, and the manipulation of the symbols according to the rules of the system. The resulting transformations are translated back into the language of the data, and the relationship discovered by the manipulations are compared with the empirical data." (Griffiths, p. 44)

Note here, however, the difficulty of "manipulating symbols" unless , for example, one is trying to explain anything other than present social developments. To seek to determine those that occurred in history, one would be well advised initially to attempt to estimate the strength of each conceivable influence that might have caused a past social occurrence or historical phenomenon.

By now governmental, educational, and commercial agencies and organizations should be able to argue convincingly that sport is a "relatively homogeneous substance" that can serve at least reasonably well as an indispensable balm or aid to human fulfillment within an individual life (adapted from Barzun [speaking about art], 1974, p. 12). However, the idea of "sport and developmental physical activity for all" on a lifelong basis continues to receive more "lip support" than actual investment based on the monetary input of government toward overall fitness and physical recreational involvement for the general population. Yet the logical argument that--through the process of total psycho-physical involvement--sport provides highly desirable "flow experience" may well be true. The question is "for whom does the bell toll?" (Csikszentmihalyi, 1993, p. 183).

Below you will find "A Model for Sport Management Development (Including a Competency-Based Approach)" (see Figure 1 below) This model is an effort to resolve the relationship between what has been called the disciplinary aspects and those aspects that have been designated as "professional" in nature. I have included five elements as the fundamental ones in a model that portrays the basic elements of the developing sport management profession.

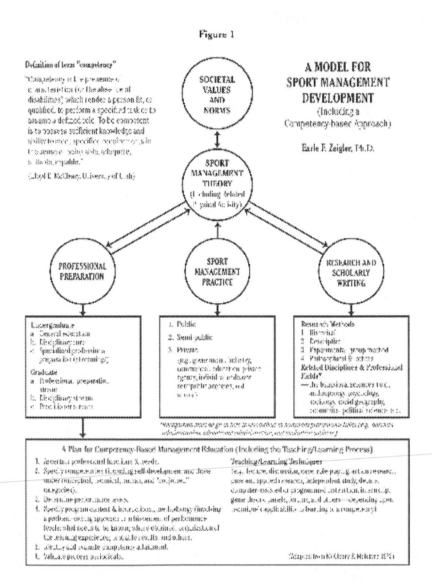

Figure 1

(Note: As it happens, these "elements" also describe the basic elements of *any* profession earlier; see Zeigler, 1972.)

The idea of competency and skill-acquisition into the model based on the recommendation by Lloyd McCleary, formerly of the University of Illinois, C-U. I subsequently realized that this entire model configuration fits very well into a description of the ongoing status of the sport-management profession.

The inclusion of "Societal Values & Norms" as an overarching entity in the model is based on the sociologic theory that the value system (i.e., the values and the norms) of a culture will be realized eventually within the society--if all goes well! Values represent the highest echelon of the social system level of the entire general action system. These values may be categorized into such "entities" as artistic values, educational values, social values, sport values, etc. Of course, all types or categories of values must be values held by personalities. The social values of a particular social system are those values that are conceived of as representative of the ideal general character that is desired by those who ultimately hold the power in the system being described. The most important social values in North America, for example, have been (1) the rule of law, (2) the socio-structural facilitation of individual achievement, and (3) the equality of opportunity (Johnson, 1994).

Norms--not to be confused with values--are the shared, sanctioned rules that govern the second level of the social structure. The average person finds it difficult to separate in his or her mind the concepts of values and norms. Keeping in mind the examples of values offered immediately above, some examples of norms are (1) the institution of private property, (2) private enterprise, (3) the monogamous, conjugal family, and (4) the separation of church and state.

Put simply, this means that decisions regarding the development of a profession are based on the prevailing values and norms over and above any scientific and/or scholarly evidence that may become available to strengthen existing theory. Fundamentally, there is a hierarchy of control and conditioning that operates within the culture that exerts pressure downward affecting all aspects of the society. (Keep in mind that this pressure may be exerted upward as well.)

Moving downward from the top of Figure 1, the second phase of the model is called "Sport Management Theory." This is the systematic arrangement of proven facts or knowledge about a professional field (or discipline in the case of a subject-matter). From such theory we can also derive assumptions and testable hypotheses that should soon amplify as a result on ongoing scholarship, research, and experience. In the process scholars and researchers will also clarify a developing (and presumably) coherent group of general and specific propositions arranged as ordered generalizations) that can be used as principles of explanation for the phenomena that have been observed. Obviously, any profession must have a sound under girding body of knowledge if it hopes to survive with its professional status fully recognized in society. Unfortunately. at present there is no such inventory of scholarly and research findings about sport management theory readily available for those involved in sport management practice, professional preparation, and research and scholarly writing contributing to disciplinary development.

Moving downward once again, the model now expands both downward and to the right and left so that there is a total of three circles. In a sense these three circles would typically "feed" or "draw" knowledge and information from the middle circle above designated as "Sport Management Theory." Note that there are arrows going backward and forward in all directions to explain necessary "reciprocity" among these entities. These arrows show the complexity of the evolving subject.

The circle on the left is designated as "Professional Preparation." It includes the planned program designed to educate the professional practitioner, the teacher of practitioners, and--arguably--the scholar and/or researcher about the subject of professional preparation. The undergraduate program would presumably include (1) general education, (2) a disciplinary core, and (3) specialized professional preparation (conceivably with streaming possibilities). The graduate program could conceivably contain three distinct streams: (1) a professional-preparation stream; (2) a disciplinary stream. and (3) a practitioner stream.

The second of the three circles alongside each other in the upper half of the model is titled "Sport Management Practice." This would include those professional practitioners with degree programs involving general education, a sport management disciplinary-base, and specialized knowledge about the theory and practice of sport management in the range of public, semipublic, and private agencies and programs involved with varying types of sport and physical activity programs.

The third of the three circles (on the right) has been given the title of "Research and Scholarly Writing." Such research knowledge and scholarly writing is developed on an ongoing basis employing existing research methods and techniques to gather knowledge (i.e. propositions of fact) about the subject of sport management at all levels and under all conditions). Such research and scholarly writing is typically carried out by university professors and qualified professionals wherever employed. Obviously, there has been great--continuing!--help in the past provided by scholars and researchers in related disciplines and professional fields (e.g., the behavioral sciences and business administration).

The Next Step for the Sport Management Profession

Now that we have had a look at where sport management has been, and where it is currently, where should it go from here? The obvious answer would appear to be to build on--i.e., add scholarly sport management literature--to the available inventory of completed research on physical education and athletics management that has been made ready for entry into both departmental and personal data banks and/or retrieval systems by the efforts of scholarly people in the field since the mid-1920s. This historical literature has been delineated and recorded for sport and physical education management.

As it exists, it can be stored in such a way that an ongoing data base can be originated, maintained, and developed. To this should be added as soon as possible the results of investigations reported in the Journal of Sport Management and similar publications worldwide (e.g., the International Journal of Sport Management). This is the bare minimum that should be carried out by someone or some group on behalf of . If completed, when professors or graduate students contemplate further research, they could at least determine what research has already been carried out on the particular topic at hand being considered for further research.

Despite the fact that this embryonic inventory of completed research is now available for easy storage and retrieval in a database, what we have been able to accomplish with this data represents merely a "scratching of the surface." So much more needs to be done by our scholars in sport and related physical activity. Presently, practitioners have been "overwhelmed" by periodical literature, monographs, and books from our field, from the allied professions, and from the related disciplines. Much of this information is interesting and valuable. However, it is so often not geared to the interests of professionals who are fulfilling many duties and responsibilities in the various positions they hold. Also, there is undoubtedly much overlapping material emanating also from the allied professions (notably recreation and park administration). Further, much of the available material--when a person by intent or chance happens to discover it--may be unintelligible, partially understandable, or not available in its essence and in a condensed form to the professional in sport management. Thus, one can only conjecture in what form such information will (or unfortunately won't) be conveyed to the many legislative or advisory boards on whose behalf we are carrying out our endeavor.

To make matters worse, because of provinciality and assorted communication barriers, our field is missing out on important findings now becoming available in Dutch, German, Japanese, Chinese, Italian, and the Scandinavian languages. Further, in addition to the above reason, because of a plethora of rules, regulations, and stipulations, people may not be receiving information about substantive reports of various government agencies at all levels. Such reports should become part of personal and departmental retrieval systems of those carrying out scholarly work in sub-disciplinary and sub-professional areas of investigation.

Interestingly, Joo and Jackson (2002) analyzed scholarly literature that had appeared in the *Journal of Sport Management* since its inception in 1987. Their analysis of 242 articles published showed that, although Trevor Slack's study in 1996 revealed that 65% of the published articles involved the delivery of either physical education or athletics programs, the emphases in research had shifted in the 1990s to marketing studies. More recently, however, there was a move to the area of organizational behavior. The results of research published in the *Journal of Sport Management,* as well as in the more recent *International Journal of Sport Management* should be entered into our bibliography and inventory as soon as possible. These findings should be correlated with studies reported as part of Zeigler's (1995) and Baker's (1983 and 1995) ongoing thesis and dissertation project with Collins and Zarriello, respectively. (Note: Contact author at <zeigrog@axion.net> to have bibliographic data from 1925-1972 downloaded.)

It is true that bibliographies of scholarly publications are occasionally made available. Further, printouts of bibliographies on specific concepts or uniterms can sometimes be purchased commercially. However, a bibliography is just that--a bibliography. Such a listing is typically not annotated to any degree, and one can hardly recall the last time a thorough bibliographical *commentary* on a topic related to sport management has been published.

The Most Important Point: The Need for an Ongoing Inventory. Still further-- and this is really the most important point--it can be argued that the profession simply does not know where it stands in regard to the steadily developing body of knowledge in the many sub-disciplinary and sub- professional aspects of sport management (e.g., sport ethics, sport law, sport economics, sport marketing). Our profession--any profession for that matter!- -needs such information as an inventory to form the basis--the theory, intellectual "underpinning," evidence, body of knowledge--for an evolving professional (practitioner's) handbook. In our case it would immediately become an essential component of every person's professional practice in the field of sport management. Nowhere does our professionals (and scholars, also) have such a steadily evolving "Inventory of Scholarly, Scientific Findings Arranged as Ordered Principles or Generalizations" in their hands (and also online) as an ever-evolving professional handbook to help them in their work daily--be they general manager, ticket manager, marketer, athletic director, head coach, management scholar or researcher, or whatever. Such information is obviously vitally important to the professional practitioner who could make use daily of the essence of this proposed "action-theory marriage." If such an inventory were to be made available, the profession should then carry such an inventory forward on a yearly, 2-, 3-, or 5-year basis of renewal for all practitioners in the profession. This deficiency can--and indeed must--be rectified as we move on into the 21st century.

Formulation of an Inventory of Scientific Findings. This recommendation to develop an inventory of scientific findings about sport management would not be unique to this field. Bernard Berelson and Gary Steiner (1964) postulated such an inventory 42 years ago in what they called the behavioral sciences. In their publication, *Human behavior: An inventory of scientific findings*, the editors and associates reported, integrated, assessed, and classified "the results of several decades of the scientific study of human behavior (p. 3). The basic plan of this formidable undertaking is fundamentally sound; thus, many of their ideas concerning format could be employed in the development of a scientific inventory of findings about sport management. Actually, it could well be carried out in all of the world's existing disciplines and then updated at regular intervals on a worldwide basis in one or more agreed-upon languages. Of course, varying emphases and certain significant differences might be introduced, but the basic approach is still valid. Berelson and Steiner summarized their task as the development of "important statements of proper generality for which there is some good amount of scientific evidence" (p. 5).

How the Inventory Would Be Constructed. The type of inventory recommended would develop through the combined effort of people in the various aspects of sport management and related disciplines and professions. The goal would be to present an inventory of knowledge on the subject of sport management--that is, to assess the present state of knowledge and scholarly thought. Thus, those who prepare this information would be writing as reporters and knowledge-integrators, presenting what they know, and what they think they know, based on the available evidence. Every effort would have to be made to avoid presenting what they hope will be known.

> (Note: Down through the years there appear to have been frequent occasions in many professions where this latter approach has been followed, intentionally or otherwise, where people make declarative statements arguing that such thoughts are indeed based on documented evidence.)

In such an inventory, the reader would find series of verified findings, principles and/or generalizations in an ordered 1-2-3-4 arrangement, typically with the citation of sources that generated the information. For example, several general theoretical propositions relative to "organizational behavior" could be considered according to several categories from Berelson and Steiner. The following findings about "The Organization," arranged as ordered generalizations, have been extracted from Berelson & Steiner (1964, pp. 365-373):

> A1 The larger, the more complex, and the more heterogeneous the society, the greater the number of organizations and associations that exist in it.
>> A1,1 Organizations tend to call forth organizations: If people organize on one side of an issue, their opponents will organize on the other side.
>> A1.2 There is a tendency for voluntary associations to become more formal.
> A2 There is always a tendency for organizations (of a nonprofit character) to turn away, at least partially, from their original goals.

A2.1 Day-to-day decisions of an organization tend to be taken as commitments and precedents, often beyond the scope for which they were initially intended, and thus they come to affect the character of the organization.

The following theory relating to the athletic director in a university-- that is, assumptions or testable hypotheses--might be included in an inventory:

1. That the manner in which the director of athletics leads his/her program is determined more by existing regulations of the educational institution itself, and the expectations of coaches and staff, than the manager's own personality and character traits.
2. That a director of athletics will find it most difficult to shift the department away from established norms.
3. That a director of athletics will receive gradually increasing support from coaches and staff members to the extent that he/she makes it possible for them to realize their personal goals.
4. That a director of athletics attempting to employ democratic leadership will experience difficulty in reaching his/her own personal goals for the program if there are a significant number of authoritarian personalities in it (adapted from Berelson & Steiner, pp. 341-346).

In reporting the available material, the language used should be as free as possible from scientific jargon. It should be understandable to the intelligent lay person and, of course, to professional practitioners in the area of sport and physical activity management. This would be difficult, because the findings would range from sport marketing to sport ethics to management competencies in a field that includes many areas of specialization. In any case, what would be presented is currently not available elsewhere in this form. This involves more than delineating by descriptive research technique what might be called "sport management literacy" (see, for example, Zeigler [1994] that presents "physical education and sport foundations" from which certain generalizations as explained above might be drawn). This type of inventory would represent a truly significant contribution to the profession of sport management, as well as the public for whose benefit sport is presumed to serve as a social institution.

To clarify this process further, the reader should understand that it may be necessary to select a particular study for inclusion in the inventory from among similar items available in the sport management literature--and also from among studies carried out in closely related fields (e.g., management science) that have a direct bearing on the major topic at hand The knowledge integrator or synthesizer (i.e. a *qualified* analyst) would be looking primarily for theory, findings, principles, generalizations, and propositions that apply to this field (i.e., the management of sport in its various forms worldwide). After accepting a finding for inclusion, it would be necessary to condense it and similar findings to one distinct principle or generalization. Next, the investigator would organize the material into subheadings that could subsequently be arranged in a logical, coherent, descending manner (e.g., Proposition A1, then A1.1, A1,1a, A1.1b, A1,1c, etc., depending upon the complexity of the proposition at hand). Finally, the resultant material would be reviewed and analyzed in order to eliminate certain technical language that might only confuse the majority of professionals for whom the inventory is primarily intended.

The goal of this project would be an inventory representing a distillation of the literature relating to the management of sport in all its forms, one that would communicate what scholars believe is known about the field to those professionals who are not specialists in the specific sub-disciplinary or sub-professional area described. This is not to say, of course, that such an inventory could not be helpful to the specialist in his or her own specialty. Further, to some extent there would at first be reliance on secondary summaries of the available literature, but this should be kept to a minimum. However, such reliance would be necessary because of the great bulk and variety of material. Also, the investigators could obtain the benefit of the evaluative judgment of the specialist who may have originally developed a summary or evaluation. Such material would be temporarily helpful in those instances where gaps in the field's own literature still exist (of which there are undoubtedly many).

Then, too, as more evidence is forthcoming, it would provide a base for improved professional operation as the fundamental and specialized management theory grows broader and deeper. Even then, the scholar, as well as the professional user of the generalized theory, would appreciate the necessity of using some qualifying statements in the development of ordered principles or generalizations (e.g., "under certain circumstances"). This inventory could be made available as an evolving professional handbook on the assumption that a steadily growing body of scientific findings about the management of developmental physical activity in sport and exercise is needed now by the many professionals in the field--be they managers, supervisors, teachers, coaches, or researchers in public, semipublic, or private agencies.

Concluding Statement

In offering this perspective to the field of sport management, Daniel Wren's cautionary thought was in my mind. In the epilogue of his outstanding *History of Management Theory and Practice* (2005), he stated: "Management is more than an economic activity, however; it is a conceptual task that must mold resources into a proper alignment with the economic, technological, social, and political facets of its environment. We neglect the 'social facets' at our peril!"

It is these very "social facets" of the enterprise that the field of sport management needs to consider more carefully in the twenty-first century. Sport, as all other social institutions, is inevitably being confronted by the need to become truly responsible. Many troubling and difficult decisions, often ethical in nature, will have to be made as the professor of sport management continues the development of this profession/discipline as it seeks to prepare those who will guide sport in the years ahead. The fundamental question facing the profession is: "What *kind* of sport should the profession promote to help shape what sort of world in the 21st century? Professional sport management societies need to decide to what extent they wish to be involved with all types of sport for all types of people of all ages as they take part in healthful sport and physical activity promoted by public, semipublic, or private agencies.

There is no doubt but that the field of sport management made great strides in the closing years of the twentieth century. Nevertheless I believe that the field--both the profession and its related disciplinary effort--must develop underlying management thought, theory, and practice in an ongoing manner to support its professional practitioners. I stress again that practitioners "on the fire line" daily in sport management should be provided with an evolving inventory of ordered generalizations as to the best ways of carrying out their endeavor.

Finally, whatever decisions are made in regard to the future, we must continue to make all possible efforts to place professional preparation for administrative or managerial leadership within our field on a gradually improving, sound, academic basis. The question of leadership confronts us from a number of different directions. Our field, and undoubtedly many others, desperately needs a continuing supply of first-class leaders. Any organization or enterprise soon begins to falter and even to stumble if it doesn't have good leadership. We should maintain our efforts to find more fine people who will take charge in the behaviorally oriented, sport management environment of today's world.

References

Baker, J. A. W., & Collins, M. S. (1983). *Research on administration of physical education and athletics 1971-1982*: A retrieval system. Reseda, CA: Mojave.

Baker, J. A. W. & Zarriello, J. (1995). *A bibliography of completed research and scholarly endeavor relating to management in the allied professions (1980-1990 inclusive)*. Champaign, IL: Stipes.

Barzun, Jacques. *The use and abuse of art.* Princeton: Princeton University Press, 1974, pp. 123-150.

Berelson, B., & Steiner, G. A. (1964). *Human behavior; An inventory of scientific findings.* New York: Harcourt, Brace & World.

Booth, F. W., & Chakravarthy, M. V. (2002). Cost and consequences of sedentary living: New battleground for an old enemy. *Research Digest (PCPFS)*, 3(16), 1-8.

Chalip, L. (2006). Toward a distinctive sport management discipline. *Journal of Sport Management*, 20(1), 1-22.

Corbin, C. B. & Pangrazi, R. P. (2001). Toward a uniform definition of wellness: A commentary. *President's Council on Physical Fitness and Sports Research Digest*, 3, 15, 1-8.

Costa, C. A. (2005). The status and future of sport management: A Delphi study. *Journal of Sport Management*, 19(2), 117-143.

Csikszentmihalyi, M. (1993), *The evolving self: A psychology for the third millennium.* NY: HarperCollins.

Encarta World English Dictionary, The. (1999). NY: St. Martin's Press.

Frisby, W. (2005). The good, the bad, and the ugly. *Journal of Sport Management*, 19(1), 1-12.

Griffiths, D. E. (1959) *Administrative Theory.* NY: Appleton-Century-Crofts.

Hahm, C.H., Beller, J. M., & Stoll, S. K. (1989). *The Hahm-Beller Values*

Choice Inventory. Moscow, Idaho: Center for Ethics, The University of Idaho.

Johnson, H. M. (1994). Modern organizations in the Parsonsian theory of action. In A. Farazmand (Ed.), *Modern organizations: Administrative theory in contemporary society* (p. 59). Westport, CT: Praeger.

Joo, J. & Jackson, E. N. (2002). A content analysis of the Journal of Sport Management:: An analysis of sport management's premier body of knowledge. *Research Quarterly for Exercise and Sport*, 73(1, Suppl.), A111.

Journal of Sport Management. (A special issue of the journal was devoted to the question of sport management research. Dated October, 2005, Vol. 19, No. 4 was titled "Expanding Horizons: Promoting Critical and Innovative Approaches to the Study of Sport Management".)

Kavussanu, M. & Roberts, G. C. (2001). Moral functioning in sport: An achievement goal perspective. *Journal of Sport and Exercise Psychology*, 23, 37-54.

Lumpkin, A., Stoll, S., & Beller, J. M. (1999). *Sport ethics: Applications for fair play* (2nd ed.). St. Louis, MO: McGraw-Hill.

Malina, R. M.. (2001). Tracking of physical activity across the life span. *Research Digest (PCPFS)*, 3-14, 1-8.

Marx, L. (1990). Does improved technology mean progress? In Tcich, A. H. (Ed.), *Technology and the future*. NY: St. Martin's Press.

National Association for Sport and Physical Education. (2001). The coaches code of   conduct. *Strategies*, 15(2), 11.

Priest, R. F., Krause, J. V., & Beach, J. (1999). Four-year changes in college athletes'   ethical value choices in sports situations. *Research Quarterly for Exercise and   Sport*, 70(1), 170-178.

Randolph, E. (2006). The big, fat American kid crisis…And 20 things we should do about it. *The New York Times*. (see: http://select.nytimes.com/2006/05/10/opinion/10talkingpoints.html?pagewanted=all).

Rudd, A., Stoll, S. K., & Beller, J. M. (1999). Measuring moral and social character among a group of Division 1A college athletes, non-athletes, and ROTC   military students. *Research Quarterly for Exercise and Sport*, 70 (Suppl. 1), 127.

Sage, G. H. (1998). Sports participation as a builder of character? *The World and I*, 3,   629-641.

Spencer, H. (1949) *Education: intellectual, moral, and physical*. London: Watts.

Steinhaus, A. H. (1952). Principal principles of physical education. In *Proceedings of the College Physical Education Association*. Washington, DC: AAHPER, pp. 5-11.

175

Stoll, S. K. & Beller, J. M. (1998). *Sport as education: On the edge*. NY: Columbia University Teachers College.

Wilcox, R. C. (1991). Sport and national character: An empirical analysis. *Journal of Comparative Physical Education and Sport.*, XIII(1), 3-27.

Wren, D. A. (2005). *The history of management thought*. NJ: John Wiley & Sons.

Zeigler, E. F. (1972). A model for optimum professional development in a field called "X." In *Proceedings of the First Canadian Symposium on the Philosophy of Sport and Physical Activity*. Ottawa, Canada: Sport Canada Directorate, pp. 16-28.

Zeigler, E. F. & Spaeth, M. J. (1975). *Administrative theory and practice in physical education and athletics*. Englewood Cliffs, NJ: Prentice-Hall.

Zeigler, E. F. (1976). In sport, as in all of life, man should be comprehensible to man. *Journal of the Philosophy of Sport*, III, 121-126

Zeigler, E. F. (ed. & au.). (1994). *Physical education and kinesiology in North America: Professional and scholarly foundations*. Champaign, IL: Stipes.

Zeigler, E. F. (1995). *A selected, annotated bibliography of completed research on management theory and practice in physical education and athletics to 1972 (including a background essay)*. Champaign, IL: Stipes.

Zeigler, E. F. (2003). Sport's plight in the postmodern world: Implications for the sport management profession," *International Journal of Sport Management*, 4(2), 93- 109.

Zeigler. E. F. (2005). *History and status of American physical education and educational sport*. Victoria, BC: Trafford.

Chapter 19
Broadening the Vision of the Sport Manager

The main problem of this investigation was to develop a means of analysis that would serve to broaden both the *professional* vision and the *personal* perspective of career managers in the field of sport management.1 The plan was to carry this out in such a way that the purpose would be accomplished by an explanation of human and natural (or physical) ecologic interaction. To achieve this goal or purpose of the study, the following five sub-problems (phrased as questions) were considered:

1. Ecology, and why sport managers should understand its various ramifications for humankind?

2. Systems analysis coordination with human and natural ecologic interaction as applied to the *organizational* "task?" of sport managers?

3. Systems analysis coordination with human and natural ecological interaction as applied to the *personal* development of sport managers?

4. Merging these interactions to achieve both *successful professional* life and a *fulfilling personal* life?

The Ramifications of Ecology for Humankind

For this analysis, ecology was defined as "the field of study that treats the relationships and interactions of human beings and other living organisms with each other and with their natural (or physical) environment" (Hawley, 1986, p. 2). Ecology, which is much more than so-called "environmentalism," is about truly understanding relationships with and/or interactions between humans and other organisms within the environment. This involvement has no doubt been with humankind over the centuries. In addition, the apparent continuing lack of understanding and full appreciation of it by leaders, not to mention all others, has still not been overcome. Further, the steadily increasing size of the world's population and the accompanying vast societal development has exacerbated the problem even further.

To put the matter more simply, the basic underlying issue of dwindling supply and increasing demand has never been brought home sufficiently to the world's leadership, much less to the majority of the people. And, in the relatively few cases where it has, urgent present need has almost invariably thrust the need for preparation to meet impending future disasters aside. In fact, that appears to be exactly what is happening this very day.

Despite the ever-increasing importance of this subject to humankind, somehow the vital importance of the subject of ecology as a fundamental social institution such as economics, politics, etc. did not begin to receive serious attention by at least a segment of society until the early 1960s. Today, however, selected countries and certain groups within these countries are striving to come to grips with the need to face up to the headlong collision looming between ecology and economics as conflicting social forces. For example, Epstein (1997) reported recently that "five years after 10,000 diplomats from 178 countries pledged to clean up the world at the United Nations-sponsored Rio Earth Summit, the first formal assessment of that pledge begins today" (March 13). At the same session, Maurice Strong, the 1992 conference chair, stated that "the process of deterioration has continued. . . ."

In 1970, Zeigler realized the problem of ecology was here to stay. So it, too, was considered as a persistent problem to the field of sport and physical activity in the same way as he had identified the five other basic social forces (or influences) of values, politics, nationalism, economics, and religion (Zeigler, 1964). No longer, as it had almost always been possible in the past, could people simply move elsewhere to locate another abundant supply of game to hunt, water to drink, or mineral resources to exploit when present resources are depleted. Today, as this problem is gradually being recognized globally, the time is past due when the field of sport and physical activity management to also pay special attention to this social force in the various aspects of its work.

More specifically, there are several very important reasons right now for the field to show ever-greater awareness of human ecologic interaction with its many ramifications for humankind. First, the promotion and subsequent development of such an awareness should soon result in the field's general acceptance of an overall human and natural (physical) ecologic orientation that could be designed to underlie all of its professional efforts. Such awareness and subsequent orientation would call the profession's attention to the fact that our basic concern as managers should be with the total life cycle of people considered both individually and collectively.

Second, the graduates of professional training programs, who subsequently serve as managers in organizations of all types functioning in culturally influenced environments, need to be so prepared they they will understand and be committed to the application of an overall ecological approach in their work. In this context this means that they, as sport management professionals, would have a basic responsibility to develop and strengthen their particular organization or collectivity in which they serve so that it will have an ongoing capability to adapt successfully to the changing (natural and cultural) environment in which it is located.

Keep in mind that fundamental changes in society are continually taking place and are accordingly influencing the profession of sport management positively, negatively, or possibly not at all. This means that, at the practitioner's level, sport managers must be ever be ready to meet such change (or lack of it) directly and adapt to it successfully. For example, cutback management or management in decline are approaches often called on in today's rapidly shifting environment. Even a reasonably basic understanding of change process itself could serve all sport managers well.

Using Systems Analysis to Explain Human and Natural Ecologic Interaction to the *Organizational* Task of Sport Managers?

The scope of the systems function in management today has gone far beyond the dreams of the "scientific management" pioneers such as Taylor, the Gilbreths, and Henri Fayol. Today the sport management profession should be fully aware of the potentialities of an ongoing systems analysis approach. Such an approach should be coordinated with the best type of overall human and natural (physical) ecologic interaction as the profession seeks to serve the public professionally through the medium of sport and physical activity. Concurrently, in this analysis of the professional function (i.e., organizational "task") of the manager, the same systems-approach concept can be merged with overall human ecologic interaction as applied to the sport manager's personal development.

The first consideration here is with the intricacies of a systems approach that give attention to how this can be done most efficiently. The assumption behind a systems approach to human and natural ecologic interaction is that the sport and physical activity-delivery organization and its manager(s)--and the people functioning within it as associates--should all understand the importance and ramifications of a complete ecological approach and be committed to its implementation in all aspects of their work. If this were understood fully, they would then strive to serve their clients and constituents in ways that help the organization grow and develop. (At this point there will not be an explanation of why the sport manager should strive for general aims in an ever-changing human and natural environment, or what specific objectives might be subsumed under these long range aims.)

With such an approach to management, the managerial team and key associated personnel would seek to develop, employ, and maintain power and influence that lead to the achievement of planned (immediate) objectives en route to long-range aims or goals. In doing so, they should involve many people within the organization in one way or another in assisting with the implementation of the fundamental processes of planning, organizing, staffing, directing, and controlling the operation of the organization (Mackenzie, 1969, pp. 80-87). Throughout this series of experiences it is imperative that good human relations be employed by all through the use of effective and efficient communication techniques.

The major responsibilities of sport managers, presuming they live up to the approved code of ethics of the North American Society for Sport Management, should include:

(1) the professional's obligations as a sport manager to actually provide services to all in society who want and need them;

(2) the professional's specific obligations to his/her clients as individuals;

(3) the professional's responsibilities to his/her employers/employing organization;

(4) the professional's obligations to his colleagues/peers and to the profession; and

(5) the professional's responsibility to overall society itself (NASSM, 1996, pp. 1-3).

All of these obligations were deliberately included in the code of ethics of the North American Society for Sport Management along with a procedure for disciplinary action to guarantee the enforcement of these responsibilities. (The latter procedure has not been enforced yet.) It should be recognized that several professions at least make some effort today to discipline those colleagues who are reported as having acted unprofessionally and unethically. If a professional person acts *illegally* within a given legal jurisdiction, it can, of course, be expected that the political jurisdiction itself will judge the severity of such action and make an appropriate decision. Such a decision will subsequently give guidance to a professional society's committee on ethics as to any disciplinary action it should take.

In meeting these basic professional obligations, the sport and physical activity manager will be involved *both* professionally and personally in an ongoing struggle for recognition and accompanying status as he/she fulfills (1) those important obligations that relate to his/her *professional life*, as well as (2) those obligations that are required for optimum *personal development*. Moving on, it will now be shown first how a schematic, systems-analysis model can assist the manager to comprehend he scope and intent of these obligations and/or responsibilities in both "realms" of his or her existence.

In the early 1970s, a schematic model for the management process was developed (the elements of the set, so to speak) that arranged the elements of a systems approach logically within a behavioral science perspective (Milstein and Belasco, 1973). The concern was with *input, thruput,* and *output,* and it was stressed that these three aspects must be strongly interrelated because any systems *outputs* "that result from transforming the human and material resources within the educational system must be at least minimally acceptable to environmental groups and organizations" (p. 81). If the outputs are not acceptable, the external groups and organizations will quite simply let it be known in short order that the "lifeline" of human and material resources will be sharply cut or eliminated.

A schematic model of such a systems model is offered here, in this case a systems model for managerial effectiveness with a professional training program for sport and physical activity managers. Here the goal or output for the purpose of this discussion is related to the education of people for various careers relating to our field. It is a substantive adaptation of the material available in both Milstein and Belasco (1973) and George (1972). (See Figure 1 below.)

Figure 1
A Systems Analysis of Human Ecologic Interaction
for the Task of the Sport and Physical Activity Manager

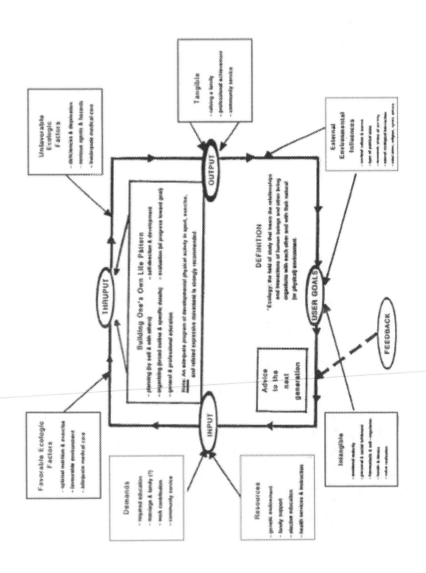

One definition of management states that it involves the execution of managerial acts by a competent person, including the application of personal, interpersonal, conceptual, technical, and conjoined skills, while combining varying degrees of planning, organizing, staffing, directing (i.e., leading), and controlling (i.e., evaluation) within the management process to assist an organization to achieve its goals effectively and efficiently (Zeigler and Bowie, 1995, p. 115).

Further, the assumption is that such managerial acts will be directed toward individual and group goals within both the internal and external environments of an organization. In this example (Fig. 1), those directing the professional training program within a college or university perceive certain societal demands and/or needs (e.g., a societal demand for various types of sport and physical activity managers). Depending on the specific circumstance, the university and its alumni and supporters respond by making available (initially or potentially) (1) material and human resources such as available capital, (2) some level of achievement in sport competition and fitness promotion, and (3) a management program staff of good, bad, or indifferent stature. All of this initial development is, of course, ultimately part of the total management process itself. After the initial input stage has been started, we are really describing functions that occur within the larger management process that is typically characterized by such terms as planning, organizing, staffing, directing, and controlling (Mackenzie, 1969). For the manager to execute these functions adequately, he or she should have acquired the necessary knowledge, competencies and skills (adapted from Katz, 1974, with advice from William Penny).

(See Figure 2 on the next page.)

Figure 2
Management Process As a Schematic Model

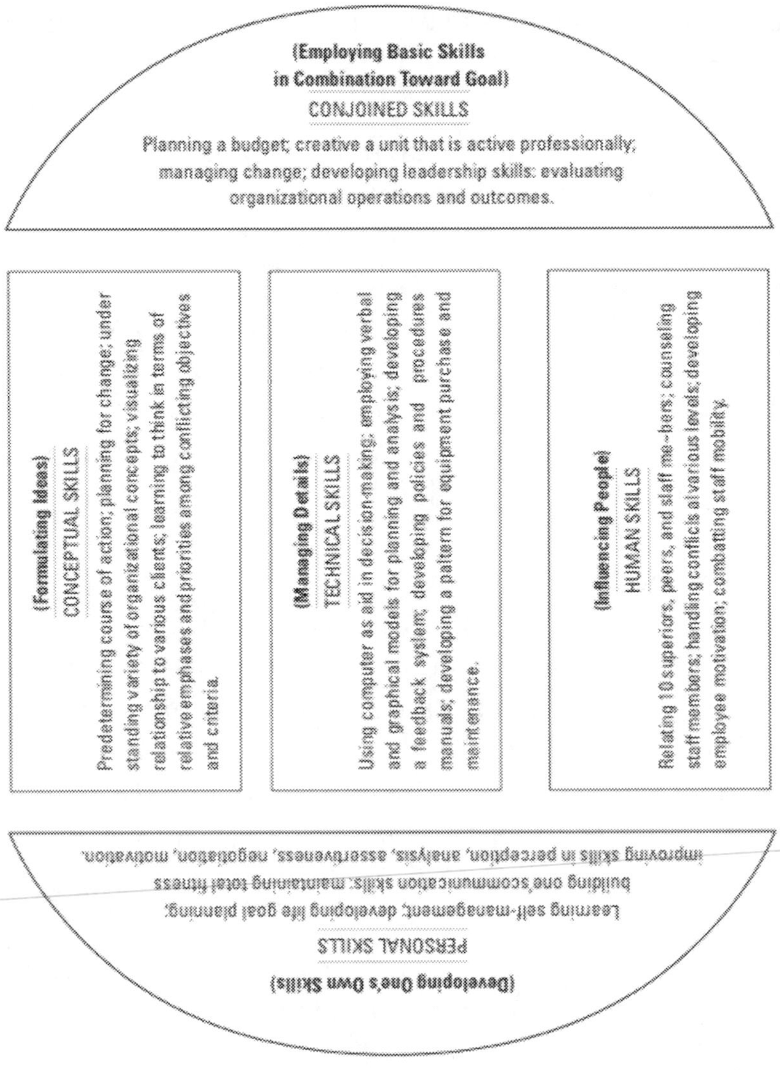

**(Employing Basic Skills
in Combination Toward Goal)**

CONJOINED SKILLS

Planning a budget; creative a unit that is active professionally;
managing change; developing leadership skills: evaluating
organizational operations and outcomes.

(Formulating Ideas)
CONCEPTUAL SKILLS

Predetermining course of action; planning for change; under standing variety of organizational concepts; visualizing relationship to various clients; learning to think in terms of relative emphases and priorities among conflicting objectives and criteria.

(Managing Details)
TECHNICAL SKILLS

Using computer as aid in decision-making; employing verbal and graphical models for planning and analysis; developing a feedback system; developing policies and procedures manuals; developing a pattern for equipment purchase and maintenance.

(Influencing People)
HUMAN SKILLS

Relating 10 superiors, peers, and staff me~bers; counseling staff members; handling conflicts al various levels; developing employee motivation; combating staff mobility

(Developing One's Own Skills)

PERSONAL SKILLS

Learning self-management; developing life goal planning;
building one's communication skills; maintaining total fitness
improving skills in perception, analysis, assertiveness, negotiation, motivation.

The names of three of the categories were taken from Katz, M. L. Skills of an effective administrator Harvard Business Review 52, 5 90-102, 1974

Management Development and Process (The knowledge and skills obtained through a competency-based approach).

Thinking of the total managerial process in this example of a system analysis model for managerial effectiveness, keep in mind that there can be three categories of parameters and/or variables that influence the entire undertaking, as follows: (1) environmental *noncontrollable* parameters (constraints or opportunities), (2) internal *controllable* variables, and (3) *partially controllable* variables (that may be external and/or internal). It is important that sport managers understand how strong these variables (influences) may be and accordingly be ever ready to factor their impact into the overall management process. Too often it appears that when such a *186*or partially controllable parameter looms suddenly on the horizon, "internal panic" results because managers--and thus their organizations, of course--have not planned ahead and typically are in no way ready for its appearance.

The environmental *noncontrollable* parameters should be viewed as external influences that must be considered seriously. They are such persistent historical problems as (1) the influence of the society's values and norms; (2) the influence of politics (the type of political state and the "stance" of the party or person in power); (3) the influence of nationalism (or whatever powerful "chauvinistic" influence might develop); (4) the influence of the prevailing economic situation (including depressions, tax increases, inflation, etc.); (5) the influence of prevailing religious groups (including boycotts, conflicting events); (6) the influence of ecology (as discussed above in this paper); and (7) the influence of competition (from other attractions, etc.).

To understand the concept of "managerial effectiveness" generally, as diagrammed in the model (Figure 1), it may help to consider specifically the relationship of managerial acts (ACTS) and the external and internal environments (Ee and Ei, respectively) of the organization to the eventual accomplishment of *at least a certain percentage* of the organization's goals (pGg) as well as *at least a certain percentage* of the (total of) individual's goals (pGi) realized. In other words, an effective manager would be a person who strives successfully to accomplish the organization's goals to the greatest possible extent, while at the same time giving adequate or ample consideration to what percentage of the goals held by individual employees is achieved. At this point, then, the concept of managerial effectiveness (Me) is added to our ongoing equation as that percentage (p) of the organization's and the (total of) individuals' goals that are realized.

(Note: Initially, the percentage of an individual's
goals achieved would be a collective percentage;

however, where individual goal achievement exists with a differentiated reward system and a varying pay scale exists, the effectiveness of any one person could be evaluated as well.)

Thus

$$Me = (pGg) + (pGi)$$

Similarly, if we accept that managerial acts (Aplanning, Aorganizing, Astaffing, etc.) are a function of a percentage (% of the attainment of) of Gg and Gi, then

$$M = F (<pGg + (pGi>)$$

Further, if G (Gg + Gi) is known, it follows that Gi) is a function of it.

(Note: For those interested, a much more detailed analysis of this mathematical model seeking to explain the management process is available in Zeigler and Bowie, 1995, pp. 115-120.)

Achieving One's *Personal* Development

We are still left with *the individual* who is involved professionally in the managerial task itself--i.e., the first-level, second-level, etc. sport and physical activity manager? Adoption of this approach would mean that this person should search for regular, ongoing opportunities for *both* personal and professional growth. This can be accomplished by implementing a similar plan that outlines a system analysis of his/her own human ecologic interaction as he or she strives *to achieve a life purpose in this profession* while concurrently serving the organization's clientele and the larger community as an informed, concerned citizen.

(See Figure 3 below)

Figure 3

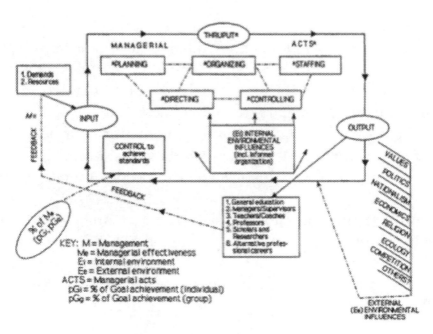

A System Analysis Model for Managerial Effectiveness
In a Professional Preparation Program for
Development Physical Activity Administrators

If this is to be carried out successfully, such a plan should also be based on a model that includes (1) *input* factors such as demands and resources; (2) *thruput* factors such as planning, evaluation, general & professional education, and evaluation; (3) tangible *output* factors such as (possibly) raising a family, professional achievement, and community service, and (4) intangible <u>user goals</u> factors such as emotional maturity, personal and social fulfillment, homeostasis and self-regulation, health & fitness, and personal & social value realization.

Basically, the discussion here outlines how sport managers can use a systems analysis approach to achieve optimal health (so-called wellness) for an effective <u>personal</u> and <u>professional</u> life within a reasonably balanced lifestyle. The idea of achieving optimal health within one's lifestyle has been equated with, and compressed in recent years by many to, the concept of "wellness.":

Wellness can be described as a lifestyle designed to reach one's highest potential for wholeness and well-being. Wellness has to do with a zest for living, feeling good about oneself, having goals and purposes for life . . . This concept is far more than freedom from symptoms of illness and basic health maintenance, but reaches beyond to an optimal level of well-being (*ERIC Digest* 3, 1986).

These thoughts and ideas are really not new, but they have been placed in a modern perspective here. Many years ago Jesse Feiring Williams defined positive health as "the ability to live best and serve most." The wellness movement has similarly recommended a balanced lifestyle. It has encouraged people to assume more responsibility for their health and to view health in the same light as Williams did earlier--that is, in a positive light in which the person's "wellness" involved all aspects of a unified organism.

In this light, the sport and physical activity manager at the input stage will typically acquire a better understanding of the demands (e.g., required education) made upon him or her, as well as an understanding of the resources (e.g., genetic endowment) necessary for a satisfactory response. (See the left section of Figure 3.)

Next, at what is called the thruput stage, the manager will appreciate more fully what steps should be taken as the individual plans, organizes, and carries out life plans. At this stage these steps should be carried out optimally through self-direction with evaluation at several strategic points along the way. (See the middle section toward the top of Figure 3.)

While all of this is taking place, there are a number of external, natural and social environmental influences impinging upon the sport manager's development (e.g., changing societal values, declining economic status; see bottom right of Figure 3.) A sport manager may have control over some of these influences, but others are often beyond control. These include both favorable and unfavorable ecologic factors. (See top right and left of Figure 3.) In the final analysis, The sport manager must make a number of crucial decisions throughout life. Such decisions may be made before the fact, so to speak, while others are made as best possible in response to natural and social factors that may often be completely or partially beyond the manager's ability to control them.

In the third or *output* stage of a sport manager's life viewed through a system analysis perspective, the manager will be asked to consider what she or he wants both her/his extrinsic, measurable and her/his intrinsic, non-measurable life goals to be. S/he will need also to seek some sort of relationship between these measurable goals and what may be called intrinsic (i.e., typically less measurable life goals). (See "tangible" output at right of Figure 3 and "intangible" output stated as "user goals" at the bottom left of Figure 3.)

In the first case, the tangible output, this refers to the person's achievement in his or her chosen career or occupation, as well as family life (however defined) and community service. In the second instance, he or she will need to assess the matter of achievement of personal and social fulfillment through the possible self-realization of those values that are felt to be most important.

(Note: A more detailed outline of this analysis of a desirable life cycle is offered below in Appendix A in this chapter.))

Finally, toward the end of this system loop, provision should be made for feedback resulting in advice to the next generation. This lifelong process for the individual is typically influenced by (1) such <u>external environmental influences</u> as (e.g.) the economic status of the society; (2) such favorable ecologic factors as (e.g.) adequate medical care; and (3) such unfavorable ecologic factors as (e.g.) the presence of noxious agents & hazards.

Achieving a Merger of *Successful Professional* Life and a *Fulfilling Personal* Life

Turning attention away from self-management (i.e., the personal life pattern of the individual sport and physical activity manager) and back to the overall organizational managerial task itself, it becomes apparent that these two managerial techniques can be merged successfully. Whether these techniques will be in any particular organization involved with the management of sport and physical activity depends on the overall management philosophy prevailing. On the surface an ecological orientation merged with a systems analysis approach to management would almost necessarily result in an "organizational management climate" that is eclectic in nature.

An "eclectic" management style may be needed because of the increasing number of situations today where a managerial team is responsible for the direction in which the organization is heading. This means that it may include, where possible and when desirable, any or all aspects of the traditional, behavioral, or decision-making patterns of managerial behavior. Thus managers may find themselves functioning with an amalgam of traditional principles, cooperative behavioralist ideas, and decisionalist competitive strategies (Gibson, Ivancevich, and Donnelly, 1997, pp. 433-439).

Concluding Statement

As the world enters the twenty-first century, such an "amalgamated" approach to professional and personal management behavior as discussed here may indeed become both necessary and desirable. This would be true so long as the original formulation of aims and objectives has occurred democratically. And, as it has happened, in Western culture people have been increasingly involved in the decision-making process in all aspects of life. As a result, an organization that fails to prepare its people adequately (i.e., both theoretically and emotionally) for the introduction of change could well find its seemingly realizable goals to be thwarted--or at least temporarily blocked--by (1) human conflicts, (2) natural or cultural barriers within the general (external), or (3) changing interpersonal and/or situational circumstances within the immediate (internal) environment (Mikalachki, A., Zeigler, E.F., & Leyshon, G.A., 1988, pp. 1-17).

In respect to the organization itself and its achievement of predetermined group and individual goals, it should be borne in mind that such organizational "growth" does not necessarily mean growth in size. This is especially important where an "ecological-oriented" business strategy has been adopted on the basis of an overall philosophical stance. It does mean that the adaptive behavior of those involved in the managerial task who (1) subscribe to an "ecological orientation" philosophically and (2) employ a systems approach functionally should be in a strong position to help *the organization* to remain viable, to be stronger, to remain competitive, and to be increasingly more effective and efficient in the accomplishment of its long range aims and immediately realizable objectives.

Finally, similar problems or obstacles of varying nature and intensity may arise within the broader general (external) environment. Of course, the hope is that such situations would serve as challenges to sport managers and their teams. The response to problems or obstacles should be heuristic in nature in the sense that a particular management team would be prepared to react to the prevailing demands and needs by adapting or possible adjusting means, behavior, and even ends at some point along the line. Sport managers should proceed only on the basis that the future belongs to those who manage effectively and efficiently in the pursuit of planned organizational goals.

References

Epstein, J. (1997). Rio Summit's promises still unfulfilled. *The Globe and Mail* (Toronto), March 13, A12.

George, C. S. (1972). *The history of management thought* (2nd Ed.). Englewood Cliffs, NJ: Prentice-Hall.

Gibson, J. I., Ivancevich, J. M., & Donnelly, J. H., Jr. (1997). *Organizations* (9th Ed.). Chicago, IL: Irwin.

Hawley, A.H. (1986). *Human ecology: A theoretical essay*. Chicago: Univ. of Chicago Press.

Katz, R.L. (Sept.-Oct. 1974). Skills of an effective administrator. *Harvard Business Review*, 51, 5:90-112.

Mackenzie, R.A. (1969). The management process in 3-D. *Harvard Education Review*, 47: 80-87.

Mikalachki, A,, Zeigler, E.F., & Leyshon, G.A. (1988). *Change process in sport and physical education management*. Champaign, IL: Stipes.

Milstein, M.M. & Belasco, J.A. (1973). *Educational administration and the bahevaioral sciences: A systems perspective*. Boston: Allyn and Bacon.

North American Society for Sport Management (NASSM). NASSM: Ethical Creed, Constitution, Operating Codes (Rev. 1996). Unpublished document.

Prevention (July 1988). High health in the middle years. 40: 7: 35-36, 38-47, 100, 105-107, 110.

Zeigler, E.F. (1964). *Philosophical foundations for physical, health, and recreation education*. Englewood Cliffs, NJ: Prentice-Hall.

Zeigler, E.F. & Bowie, G.W. (1995) *Management competency development in sport and physical education*. Champaign, IL: Stipes.

Appendix:

Employing a Systems Analysis Approach in a Quest for Optimal Health and Effective Living

INPUT Stage A: What *Demands* Are Made on a Person in Today's World?

1. Early Family Membership
2. Education
3. Marriage & Family
4. Work Contribution
5. Community Service

INPUT Stage B: What *Resources* Are Typically Provided?

1. Early Family Support
2. Educational Opportunities
3. External Social Influences
4. Employment Opportunities
5. Health & Community Services

THRUPUT Stage A: What *Steps* Should Be Taken in Developing
      One's Own Life As Fully As Possible?

1. Planning for the Long Haul Ahead
2. Organizing the Required Factors & Details
3. Implementing Life Stages Through Self-Direction
4. Evaluation of Progress Made in Goal Achievement
5. Modifying or Redirecting One's Developmental Pattern
6. Planning for Retirement

THRUPUT Stage B: What *External Environmental Factors*
      Might Be Encountered?

1. Favorable Ecologic Factors:
   a. Good Heredity; No Disabling Disease
   b.. Healthy Environment; No Debilitating Factors
   c. Safe Living; No Careless Risk
   d. Optimal Nutrition, Exercise, & Rest
   e. Challenges; Satisfying Work & Recreation
   f. Commitment to High Values
   g. Competent Medical & Dental Care
   h. Homeostasis & Self-Regulation; Emotional Maturity
   i. Personal & Social Fulfillment; Freedom & Privacy

2. Unfavorable Ecologic Factors

a. Poor Heredity; Disabling Disease
b. Unhealthy Environment; Noxious Agents & Hazards
c. Unsafe Living; Careless Risk
d. Inadequate Nutrition, Exercise, & Rest
e. Little Challenge; Unrewarding Work & Recreation
f. Lack of Commitment to High Values
g. Inadequate Medical & Dental Care
h.. Deprivation; Excesses; Immaturity
. i. Low Level of Achievement & Personal Fulfillment;
   Restraints & Overcrowding

3. Improved Health in the Middle Years (40-49)

a. Assessment of nutritional intake
(including reasonable coffee intake, compensating
for "metabolic slowdown"; watch amounts of alcohol,
desserts, and fat consumed; pare diet down & exercise)

b. Body conditioning
(work with weights; stretch; watch for "middle-age
spread"; strive for consistency, not intensity;
exercise will burn off fat)

c. Circulo-respiratory conditioning
(regular, moderate exercise within "threshold zone"
will keep heart healthy--serves to lower high blood
pressure and blood cholesterol)

d. Contraception
(continue birth-control methods for one year post-
menstrually; barrier contraceptives still recommended
for middle years; check new methods available carefully; consider clip sterilization)
e. Good sex
(sexual interest peaks for women in late 30's or early
40's; males better lovers at this stage; communication
of feelings; stay healthy; maintain strength of PC
and/or vaginal muscles; vaginal lubricants; remain
active sexually; women may consider HRT.

f. Healthy relationships
(beware of burnout and boredom; involvement in shared
tasks and interests; cultivation of friends)

g. Job transition
(change positions only for the right reasons; be more

concerned about fulfilling needs and interests than
before building size of bank account or stock
holdings; your age is biggest asset; experience
brings ability to solve practical problems)

h. Brainpower
(stay mentally active and even work for improvement;
try not to act your age; limit TV viewing time;
strive to be productive creatively; boost memory
power and pay attention.

(Note: This section above is based on "High
Health in the Middle Years," *Prevention*, July 1988).

OUTPUT Stage A: Tangible (Extrinsic) Life Accomplishments

1. A Family Raised Successfully
2. Achievement in Chosen Career
3. Record of Community Service
4. Plan Developed for Successful Retirement

OUTPUT Stage B: Intangible (Intrinsic) Life Accomplishments

1. Personal & Social Fulfillment
   Through Value Realization
2. System Feedback: Advice to the Next Generation

THE OVERALL GOAL: Optimal Health, Effective Living,
              and Personal & Social Fulfillment

Chapter 20
Sport's Challenge in the Postmodern World: Becoming "Part of the Solution"

Note: In this final chapter, some basic points made earlier will be repeated for re-emphasis.

Our thoughts turn to the "adventure" of civilization as Earth enters what is commonly termed "The 21st Century" (C.E.). Such pondering has been indelibly colored in this aftermath of September 11, 2001. Life goes on inexorably as an adventure, however, in what we like to call "developing" civilization. This opinion is based on the dictionary definition of the term as either an "exciting experience" or a "bold undertaking" (*Encarta World English Dictionary*, 1999, p. 23). Within world culture of the 20th century, competitive sport has gradually but steadily become a significant social force.

The "Adventure" of Civilization

Before considering what is here termed the "plight" of sport, recall that the adventure of civilization began technological headway at least because of now-identifiable forms of early striving which embodied elements of great creativity (e.g., the invention of the wheel, the harnessing of fire). The subsequent development in technology, slowly but steadily, offered humans some surplus of material goods over and above that needed for daily living. For example, the early harnessing of nature created the irrigation systems of Sumeria and Egypt, and these accomplishments led to the establishment of the first cities. Here material surpluses were collected, managed, and sometimes squandered; nevertheless, necessary early accounting methods were created that subsequently expanded in a way that introduced writing to the human scene. As we now know, the development of this form of communication in time helped humans expand their self-consciousness and to evolve gradually and steadily in all aspects of culture. For better or worse, however, the end result of this social and material progress has created a mixed agenda characterized by good and evil down to the present. The world's blanketing communications network has now exceeded humankind's ability to cope with it.

Muller (1952) concluded, "the adventure of civilization is necessarily inclusive" (p. 53). By that he meant that evil will probably always be with humankind to some degree, but it is civilization that sets the standards and accordingly works to eradicate at least the worst forms of such evil. Racial prejudice, for example, must be overcome. For better or worse, there are now more than six billion people on earth, and that number appears to be growing faster than a national debt! These earth creatures are black-, yellow-, brown-, or white-skinned, but fundamentally we now know from genetic research that there is an "overwhelming oneness" in all humankind that we dare not forget in our overall planning (Huxley, 1957).

As various world evils are overcome, or at least held in check, scientific and accompanying technological development will be called upon increasingly to meet the demands of the exploding population. Gainful work and a reasonable amount of leisure will be required for further development. Unfortunately, the necessary leisure required for the many aspects of a broad, societal culture to develop fully, as well as for an individual to grow and develop similarly within it, has come slowly. The average person is far from a full realization of such benefits. Why "the good life" for all has been so slow in arriving is not an easy question to answer. Of course, we might argue that times do change slowly, and that the possibility of increased leisure has really come quite rapidly--once humans began to achieve some control of their environment.

"Universal Civilization" or the Clash of Civilizations?

Naipaul (1990) theorized that we are developing a "universal civilization" characterized by (1) the sharing of certain basic values, (2) what their societies have in common (e.g., cities and literacy, (3) certain of the attributes of Western civilization (e.g., market economies and political democracy), and (4) consumption patterns (e.g., fads) of Western civilization. Samuel Huntington (1998), the eminent political scientist, doesn't see this happening, however, although he does see some merit in these arguments. He grants that Western civilization is different than any other civilization that has ever existed because of its marked impact on the whole world since 1500. However, he doesn't know whether the West will be able to reverse the signs of decay already present and thus renew itself.

Sadly, there have been innumerable wars throughout history with very little if any let-up to the present. Nothing is so devastating to a country's economy as war. Now, whether one likes it or not, the world is gradually sliding into what Huntington has designated as "the clash of civilizations." It appears that the American government in power has seized upon his analysis as a justification to move still further in the War on Terrorism by the installation of what has euphemistically been called a "modernized regime" in Iraq. It is argued that this "accomplishment" would help toward the gradual achievement of worldwide democratic values along with global capitalism and so-called free markets.

The Misreading of Huntington's Thought. This misreading of Huntington's thought, however, needs to be corrected. As it stands, he asserts, "Western belief in the universality of Western culture suffers three problems. . . .It is false; it is immoral; and it is dangerous" (p. 310). He believes strongly that these religion-based cultures, such as the Islamic and the Chinese, should be permitted to find their own way in the 21st century. In fact, they will probably do so anyhow, no matter what the West does. Then individually (hopefully not together!), they will probably each become superpowers themselves. The "unknown quality" of their future goals will undoubtedly fuel the desires of those anxious for the United States to maintain overwhelming military superiority along with continually expanding technological capability.

While this is going on, however, the United States needs to be more aware of its own internal difficulties. It has never solved its "inner-city problem," along with increases in antisocial behavior generally (i.e., crime, drugs, and violence). Certainly the decay of the traditional family (i.e., husband, wife, two children) could have long-term implications as well. Huntington refers further to a "general weakening of the work ethic and rise of a cult of personal indulgence (p. 304). Still further, there is a definite decline in learning and intellectual activity as indicated by lower levels of academic achievement creating a need for course grade "aggrandizement" (i.e., the gentleman's "C" is "history"). Finally, there has been a marked lessening of "social capital" (the amount of "volunteering" including personal trust in others to meet individual needs).

Schlesinger's Analysis of America. These conflicting postulations by Huntington and Naipaul are stated here merely to warn that the present "missionary culture" of the United States is, in many ways, not really a *true* culture anyhow. So states Arthur Schlesinger, Jr. (1998), the distinguished historian. He points out that in recent years the U.S.A. has gradually acquired an ever-increasing multi-ethnicity. In *The Disuniting of America,* he decries the present schisms occurring in the United States. He is most

197

concerned that the melting pot concept formerly so prominent in the States is becoming a "Tower of Babel" concept--just like Canada!

He understands, however, that "Canadians have never developed a strong sense of what it is to be a Canadian" by virtue of their dual heritage (p. 17). Huntington explains further that an attempt to export democratic and capitalistic values vigorously to the world's other cultures may be exactly the wrong approach. He believes that they may well be looking mainly for stability in their own traditions and identity. Japan, for example, has shown the world that it is possible to become "rich and modern" without giving up their illiberal "core identity." Struggle as all cultures do for renewal when internal decay sets in, no civilization has proven that it is invincible indefinitely. This is exactly why Muller characterized history as somehow being imbued with a "tragic sense."

The "Tragic Sense" of Life

This "tragic sense' that history has displayed consistently was described by Herbert Muller (1952), in his magnificent treatise titled *The Uses of the past* . Muller disagrees with the philosopher Hobbes (1588-1679), however, who stated in his *De homine* that very early humans existed in an individual state of nature in which life was anarchic and basically "solitary, poor, nasty, brutish, and short." Muller argued in rebuttal that life "might have been poor and short, but that it was never solitary or simply brutish" (p. 6).

Accordingly, Muller's approach to history was in the spirit of the great tragic poets, a spirit of reverence and/or irony. It is based on the assumption that the tragic sense of life is not only the profoundest, but also the most pertinent for an understanding of both past and present (p. viii).

Muller believed that the drama of human history has been characterized up to now by high tragedy in the Aristotelian sense. As he stated, "all the mighty civilizations have fallen because of tragic flaws; as we are enthralled by any golden age we must always add that it did not last, it did not do" (p. viii). This brings to mind that conceivably the 20th century of the modern era may turn out to have been the "Golden Age" of the United States. As unrealistic as this may sound because today the United States is the most powerful nation in the history of life on Earth, there could be misgivings developing about the blind optimism concerning history's malleability and compatibility in keeping with American ideals.

"The future as history." More than a generation ago, Heilbroner (1960) arrived at this position similarly. He explained in his "future as history" concept that America's belief in a personal "deity of history" may be short-lived in the 21st century. As he stated this, he emphasized the need to search for a greatly improved "common denominator of values" (p. 170) in the face of technological, political, and economic forces that are "bringing about a closing of our historic future." As the world turns today in 2002, one may laugh at this prediction. Yet, looking at the situation from a starkly different perspective even earlier, Toynbee (1947) came to a quite similar conclusion in his monumental *A Study of History* from still another standpoint. He theorized that humankind must return to the one true God from whom it has gradually but steadily fallen away. You can challenge him on this opinion, as the author (an agnostic) most assuredly does. Yet, no matter--the way things are going at present--we on the Earth had best try to use our heads as intelligently and wisely as possible. As we get on with striving to make the world as effective, efficient, and humane as possible, we need to make life as replete with *Good,* as opposed to *Evil,* as we possibly can. With this plea for an abundance of righteousness, the reader may no longer be wondering where this analysis is heading. Let us turn now to what the author terms the "plight" of sport management.

The "Plight" of Sport Management

At this point, having placed the "adventure" of civilization in some perspective, this analysis now shifts its focus to sport and related physical activity. Here is a societal institution that became an ever-more powerful social force in the 20th century. In this study the author is attempting to analyze philosophically and sociologically what the author reluctantly calls the "plight" of sport management. Basically, the argument is that society is governed by strong social forces or *institutions.* Among those social institutions are (1) the values (including norms devised thereafter) , (2) the type of political state in vogue, (3) the prevailing economic system, (4) the religious beliefs present, etc. To these longstanding institutions, the author has added the influence of such other forces as education, science and technological advancement, concern for peace, *and now sport itself.* (Zeigler, 1989, Part II). Of these, the *values,* and the accompanying norms developed, form the strongest institution of all.

Crossing the Postmodern Divide. Whether we all recognize it or not, *similar to all other professions today*, the burgeoning sport management profession is presently striving to cross what has been termed the postmodern divide. An epoch in civilization approaches closure when many of the fundamental convictions of its advocates are challenged by a substantive minority of the populace. It can be argued that indeed the world is moving into a new epoch as the proponents of postmodernism have been affirming over recent decades. Within such a milieu there are strong indications that sport management is going to have great difficulty crossing this chasm, this so-called, postmodern divide.

A diverse group of postmodern scholars argues that many in democracies, under girded by the various rights being propounded (e.g., individual freedom, privacy), have come to believe that now they too require--and deserve!--a supportive "liberal consensus" within their respective societies. Conservative, essentialist elements prevail at present and are functioning strongly in many Western political systems. With their more authoritative orientation in mind, conservatives believe the deeper foundation justifying this claim of a need for a more liberal consensus has never been fully rationalized. *However, it can be argued that postmodernists now form a substantive minority supporting a more humanistic, pragmatic, liberal consensus in which highly competitive sport is viewed as an increasingly negative influence on society* (Borgman, 1993, p. 78). If this statement has merit--there are strong indications that the present sport management profession--*as known today*--will have difficulty crossing this post-modern divide that has been postulated.

Characterizations of Competitive Sport

Having stated that "sport" has become a strong social force or institution, it is true also that there has been some ambiguity about what such a simple word means. The word "sport" is used in many different ways as a noun. The number of definitions is now 14 in the most recent *Encarta World English Dictionary* (1999, p. 1730). In essence, what is being described here is an athletic activity requiring skill or physical prowess. It is typically of a competitive nature as in racing, wrestling, baseball, tennis, or cricket. For the people involved, sport is often serious, and participants may even advance to a stage where competitive sport becomes a semi-professional or a professional career choice. For a multitude of others, however, sport is seen more as a diversion, as recreational in nature, and as a pleasant pastime.

A Social Institution Without a Theory. Viewed collectively, the author's argument here is that at present the "totality" of sport appears to have become a strong social institution--*but one that is without a well-defined theory.* This assertion may have been recognized by others too. Yet, at this point the general public, including most politicians, seems to believe that "the more competitive sport we have, the merrier!" However, those in the sport management profession ought right now to answer such questions as (1) what purposes competitive sport has served in the past, (2) what functions it is fulfilling now, (3) where it seems to be heading, and (4) how it *should* be employed to serve *all* humankind.

How Sport Serves Society. In response to these questions, without careful delineation or any priority at this point, the author is stating that sport as presently operative can be subsumed in a non-inclusive list as possibly serving in the following ways:

1. As an organized religion (for those with or without another similar competing affiliation)
2. As an exercise medium (often a sporadic one)
3. As a life-enhancer or "arouser" (puts excitement in life)
4. As a trade or profession (depending upon one's approach to it)
5. As an avocation, perhaps as a "leisure-filler" (at either a passive, vicarious, or active level)
6. As a training ground for war (used throughout history for this purpose)
7. As a "socializing activity" (an activity where one can meet and enjoy friends)
8. As an educational means (i.e., the development of positive character traits, however described)

In retrospect, the author finds it most interesting that he didn't list sport "as a developer of positive character traits" until last! He now wonders why. . . .

This listing could undoubtedly be larger. It could have included such terms as (1) sport "the destroyer," (2) sport "the redeemer," (3) sport "the social institution being tempted by science and technology," (4) sport "the social phenomenon by which heroes and villains are created," or, finally, (5) sport "the social institution that has survived within an era characterized by a vacuum of belief for many." However, the author must stop. believing this listing is sufficient to make the necessary point here.

The hope is that you, the reader, will agree that the sport manager truly needs to understand what competitive sport has become in society, as well as why a great many of its other promoters are confronted with a dilemma. The argument here is that sport too--as is true for all other social institutions--is inevitably being confronted by the postmodern divide. In crossing this frontier, many troubling and difficult decisions, often ethical in nature, will have to be made as those related to sport management in one of several ways, for example, seek to prepare or engage prospective professionals who will guide sport into becoming a responsible social institution. The fundamental question facing the profession is: *"What kind of sport does it want to promote to help shape what sort of world in the 21st century?"*

Is Sport Fulfilling Its Presumed Educational and Recreational Roles Adequately?

What implications does all of this have for sport as it enters the 21st century? *In the opinion of the author, there are strong indications that sport's presumed educational and recreational roles in the "adventure" of civilization are not being fulfilled adequately.* Frankly, the way commercialized, over-emphasized sport has been operated, it can be added to the list of symptoms of American internal decay enumerated above (e.g., drugs, violence, decline of intellectual interest, dishonesty, greed). If true, this inadequacy inevitably throws a burden on sport management as a profession to do something about it. Sport, along with all of humankind, is facing the postmodern divide.

Reviewing this claim in some detail, Depauw (*Quest*, 1997) argues that society should demonstrate more concern for those who have traditionally been marginalized in society by the sport establishment (i.e., those excluded because of sex or "physicality"). She speaks of "The (In)Visibility of DisAbility" in our culture. Depauw's position is backed substantively by what Blinde and McCallister (1999) call "The Intersection of Gender and Disability Dynamics."

A second point of contention about sport's contribution relates to the actual "sport experience." The way much sport has been conducted, the public has every right to ask, "Does sport build character or 'characters'?"

Kavussannu & Roberts (2001) recently showed that, even though "sport participation is widely regarded as an important opportunity for character development," it is also true that sport "occurs in a context that values ego orientation (e.g. winning IS the most important thing)."

Sport's ContributionToday. What is competitive sport's contribution today? Delving into this matter seriously might produce a surprise--or perhaps not. It may well be that sport is contributing significantly in the development of what are regarded as *social* values--that is, the values of teamwork, loyalty, self-sacrifice, and perseverance consonant with prevailing corporate capitalism in democracy and in other political systems as well. *Conversely,* however, it may also be that there is now a great deal of evidence that sport is developing an ideal that opposes the fundamental moral virtues of honesty, fairness, and responsibility in the innumerable competitive experiences provided (Lumpkin, Stoll, and Beller, 1999).

Significant to this discussion are the results of investigations carried out by Hahm, Stoll, Beller, Rudd, and others in the late 1980s and 1990s. The Hahm-Beller Choice Inventory (HBVCI) has now been administered to athletes at different levels in a variety of venues. It demonstrates conclusively that athletes will not support what is considered "the moral ideal" in competition. An athlete with moral character should demonstrate the moral character traits of honesty, fair play, respect, and responsibility whether an official is present to enforce the rules or not. This finding was substantiated by Priest, Krause, and Beach (1999) who reported that their findings in the four-year changes in college athlete's ethical value choices were consistent with other investigations. They showed decreases in "sportsmanship orientation" and an increase in "professional" attitudes associated with sport.

On the other hand, even though dictionaries define social character similarly, sport practitioners, including participants, coaches, parents, and officials, have come to believe that character is defined properly by such values as self-sacrifice, teamwork, loyalty, and perseverance (Rudd. 1999). The common expression in competitive sport is: "He/she showed character"--meaning "He/she 'hung in there' to the bitter end!" [or whatever]. Rudd confirmed also that coaches explained character as "work ethic and commitment." This coincides with what sport sociologists have found. Sage (1988, p. 634) explained that "Mottoes and slogans such as 'sports builds character' must be seen in the light of their ideological issues" In other words, competitive sport is structured by the nature of the society in which it occurs. This would appear to mean that over-commercialization, drug-taking, cheating, bribe-taking by officials, violence, etc. at all levels of sport are simply reflections of the culture in which we live.

Thus, we are left with sport's *presumed* relationship with moral character development that has been misinterpreted. And so, despite its claims to be "the last best hope on earth," American culture--where this "redefinition" of the term character has occurred--appears to be facing what Berman (2000) calls "spiritual death" (p. 52). He makes this claim because of "its crumbling school systems and widespread functional illiteracy, violent crime and gross economic inequality, and apathy and cynicism."

At this point, one can't help but recall that the ancient Olympic Games became so excessive with ills that the event was abolished. The Games were begun again only by the spark provided in the late 19th century by de Coubertin's "noble amateur ideal." The way things are going today, it is not unthinkable that the steadily increasing excesses of the present Olympic Games Movement could well bring about their demise again. However, they could well be only symptomatic of a larger problem confronting world culture.

This discussion about whether sport's presumed educational and recreational roles have justification in fact could go on indefinitely. So many negative incidents have occurred that one hardly knows where to turn to avoid further negative examples. On the one hand we read the almost unbelievably high standards set in the Code of Conduct developed by the Coaches Council of the National Association for Sport and Physical Education (NASPE) (2001); yet, conversely we learn that today athletes' concern for the presence of moral values in sport declines over the course of a university career (Priest, Krause, and Beach, 1999).

Sedentary Living Has Caught Up With America. With this as a backdrop, we learn further that Americans are concurrently, for example, increasingly facing the cost and consequences of sedentary living (Booth & Chakravarthy, 2002). Additionally, Malina (2001) tells us there is a need to track people's physical activity across their lifespans. North America hasn't yet been able to devise and accept a uniform definition of wellness for all people. The one thought that emerges from these various assessments is as follows: Many people give every evidence of wanting their "sport spectaculars" *for the few*-- much more than they want all people of all ages and all conditions to have meaningful sport, exercise, and physical recreation involvements throughout their lives.

In Canada, conversely, Tibbetts (2002), for example, described a most recent Environics survey that explained that "65% of Canadians would like more government money spent on local arenas, playgrounds, and swimming pools, as well as on sports for women, the poor, the disabled, and aboriginals."

Official Sport's Response to the Prevailing Situation

How does what is often called the "sport officialdom" respond to this situation? Answers to this question are just about everywhere as we think, for example, of the various types of scandals tied to both the summer and winter versions of the Olympic Games. For example, the Vancouver *Province* (2000) reported that the former "drug czar" of the U.S. Olympic Team, Dr. Wade Exum, charged that half of the team used performance-enhancing drugs to prepare for the 1996 Games. After making this statement, the response was rapid: he was forced to resign! He is currently suing the United States Olympic Committee for racial discrimination and harassment.

Viewed in a different perspective, as reported by Wallis (2002), Dr. Vince Zuaro, a longtime rules interpreter for Olympic wrestling, said recently: "Sports are so political. If you think what happened with Enron is political, [try] Olympic officiating. . . .Every time there's judging involved, there's going to be a payoff." Further, writing about the credibility of the International Olympic Committee, Feschuk (2002) stated in an article titled "Night of the Olympic Dead": "The IOC has for so long been inflicting upon itself such severe ethical trauma that its survival can only be explained by the fact that it has passed over into the undead. Its lifeless members shuffle across the globe in a zombie-like stupor, one hand extended to receive gratuities, the other held up in exaggerated outrage to deny any accusations of corruption."

At the same time, Dr. Ayotte, director of the only International Olympic Committee-accredited testing laboratory in Canada, explains that young athletes believe they *must* take drugs to compete successfully. "People have no faith in hard work and food now," she says, to achieve success in sport (Long, 2001).

Dick Pound's Reward for Distinguished Service. Closing out reference to the Olympic Games Movement, recall the case of Dick Pound, the Canadian lawyer from Montreal, who had faithfully and loyally striven most successfully to bolster the Games' finances in recent decades. He had also taken on the assignment of monitoring the situation with drugs and doping, as well as the bribery scandal associated with the Games held in Salt Lake City. In the election to succeed retiring President Samaranch, Pound unbelievably finished in third place immediately behind a man caught in a bribery scandal just a short time earlier.

Finally, in the realm of international sport, Norwegian professor Dr. Hans B. Skaset (2002), a Norwegian professor, in response to a query, emailed the author about a prediction he would be making at a conference on drugs in sport in November, 2002. He predicted as keynote speaker that:

> Top international sport will cut itself free from its historical values and norms. After working with a clear moral basis for many years, sport by 2008-2010 will continue to be accepted as a leading genre within popular culture--but not, as it was formerly, a model for health, fairness, and honorable conduct. . . .

Switching venues, you don't see hockey promoters doing anything to really curb the Neanderthal antics of professional hockey players. Considering professional sport generally, note the view of sport sociologist, Steven Ortiz, who has found in his study that "there clearly seems to be a 'fast-food sex' mentality among professional athletes" (Cryderman, 2001).

In addition, in the realm of higher education, Canadian universities are gradually moving toward the athletic-scholarship approach that certain universities in the East and Midwest sections of Canada have been following for years illegally (Naylor, 2002)! In September, 2001, a Halifax, Nova Scotia university team, the St. Mary Huskies, beat Mount Allison, a Sackville, New Brunswick university football team in the same conference, by a score of 105-0. In this article, one of a series sponsored by *The Globe and Mail* (Toronto), various aspects of this lopsided development were considered. Interestingly, funding for recruited athletes is just "penny-ante" compared to the support provided for the scholarship programs of various upper-division university conferences in the United States .

How to Reclaim Sport (Weiner). In writing about how society's obsession with sport has "ruined the game," Weiner (2000), a sportswriter with the Minneapolis Star-Tribune, asks the question: "How far back must we go to remember that sports matter?" Recalling the time when "sports had meaning," and "sports were accessible," he recommends that society can only "reclaim sports from the corporate entertainment behemoth" if it does the following:

1. Deprofessionalize college and high school sports,
2. Allow some form of public ownership of professional sport teams,
3. Make sports affordable again, and
4. Be conscious of the message sport is sending.

To summarize, sport managers at various levels of what may be called "the sport industry" have quite simply conducted themselves in keeping with the prevailing political environment and ethos of the general public. They have presumably not understood and accordingly not accepted the contention that there is an urgent need for sport to serve as a beneficent social institution with *an underlying theory* looking to humankind's betterment (an *"IF* 'this,' *THEN* 'that' will result" type of approach).

Thus, it can be argued that society does indeed believe that competitive sport is doing what it is intended to do--i.e., provide *both* non-moral and moral values to those involved. (The *non-moral* values could be listed as recognition, money, and a certain type of power, whereas the *moral* values could be of a nature designed to help the team achieve victory-- dedication, loyalty, self-sacrifice.) *If this assessment is accurate, the following question must be asked: Does the prevailing ethos in sport competition need to be altered so that this activity truly helps boys and girls, and men and women too, to learn honesty fair play, justice, responsibility, and beneficence (i.e., doing good)?*

Seemingly the only conclusion to be drawn is that the sport industry is "charging ahead" driven by the prevailing capitalistic, "global village" image of the future. Increasingly in competitive sport, such theory is embraced ever more strongly, an approach in which winning is overemphasized with resulting higher profits to the promoters through increased gate receipts. This same sport industry is aided and abetted by a society in which the majority do not recognize sufficiently the need for sport to serve as *a social institution that truly results in individual and social good.*. On the one hand there are scholars who argue that democratic states, undergirded by the various human rights legislated (e.g., equal opportunity), urgently need a supportive "liberal consensus" to maintain a social system that is fair to all. Yet, conservative, essentialist elements functioning in the same social system evidently do not see this need for a more humanistic, pragmatic consensus about the steadily mounting evidence showing a need for *ALL* people to be active physically throughout their lives.

This is a substantive aspect of the basis for the argument that commercialized sport will have great difficulty "crossing the post-modern divide." Zeigler (1996) pointed out that almost every approach to "the good life" stresses a need for an individual's relationship to developmental physical activity such as sport and fitness. Question: Should not professionals in NASSM and similar societies worldwide be assessing the social institution of sport to determine whether the way sport is presented to professional students is resulting in their becoming imbued with a desire to promote the concept of "sport for all" to foster overall human betterment?

Functioning With an Indeterminate, Muddled Theory. Once again, before considering future societal scenarios that world culture is facing, the argument should be made again that today sport is functioning vigorously with *an indeterminate, muddled theory* implyng that sport competition builds *both* "moral" *and* "social" character traits consonant with democracy and capitalism. Crossing the post-modern divide means basically also that sport and physical activity management educators should see through the false front and chicanery of the developing economic and technological facade of the global hegemony. They should see to it that their students understand this development. Face it: Sport is simply being *used* as a powerful institution in this "Brave New World" of the 21st century.

Future Societal Scenarios

Walter Truett Anderson (1997), president of the American Division of the World Academy of Art and Science, has sketched *four* different scenarios as postulations for the future of earthlings in this ongoing adventure of civilization. In this essay "Futures of the Self," taken from *The Future of the Self: Inventing the Postmodern Person* , Anderson argues convincingly that current trends are adding up to a turn-of-the-century identity crisis for humankind. The creation of the present "modern self," he explains, began with Plato, Aristotle, and with the rights of humans in Roman legal codes.

The developing conception of self bogged down in the Middle Ages, but fortunately was resurrected in the Renaissance Period described by many historians as the second half of The Middle Ages. Since then the human "self" has been advancing like a "house afire" as the Western world has gone through an almost unbelievable transformation. It appears that scientists like Galileo and Copernicus influenced philosophers such as Descartes and Locke to foresee a world in which the self was invested with human rights.

"One World, Many Universes." Anderson's (1997) "One World, Many Universes" version is the most likely to occur. This is a scenario characterized by high economic growth, steadily increasing technological progress, and globalization combined with high psychological development. Such psychological maturity, he predicts, will be possible for a certain segment of the world's population because "active life spans will be gradually lengthened through various advances in health maintenance and medicine" (pp. 251-253)

Nevertheless, a problem has developed with this dream of individual achievement of inalienable rights and privileges, one that looms large at the beginning of this new century. The *modern self* envisioned by Descartes, a rational, integrated self that Anderson likens to Captain Kirk at the command post of Starship Enterprise, appears to be having an identity crisis. The image of this bold leader (he or she!) taking us fearlessly into the great unknown has begun to fade as alternate scenarios for the future of life on Earth are envisioned. In a world where globalization and economic "progress" seemingly *must be rejected* because of catastrophic environmental concerns or "demands," the bold-future image could well "be replaced by a post-modern self; decentered, multidimensional, and changeable" (p. 50).

Captain Kirk, or "George W," as he "boldly goes where no man has gone before"--this time to rid the world of terrorists and evil leaders), is facing a second crucial change. As leaders seek to shape the world of the 21st century, based on Anderson's analysis, there is another force--the systemic-change force mentioned above--that is shaping the future. This all-powerful force may well exceed the Earth's ability to cope. As gratifying as such factors as "globalization along with economic growth" and "psychological development" may seem to the folks in a coming "One-World, Many Universes" scenario, there is a flip side to this prognosis. Anderson identifies this image as "The Dysfunctional Family" scenario. All of these benefits of so-called progress are highly expensive and available now only to relatively few of the six billion plus people on earth. Anderson foresees this as "a world of modern people happily doing their thing; of modern people still obsessed with progress, economic gain, and organizational bigness; *and of postmodern people being trampled and getting angry"* [italics added] (p. 51). As people get angrier, present-day terrorism in North America could seem like child's play.

What Kind of A World Do You Want for Your Descendants?

The ultimate question here is whether members of THE one North American professional society for sport management, along with professionals in other sport management societies worldwide, are cognizant of, and approve of, the situation as it has developed. Are we simply "going along with the crowd" while taking the path of least resistance? Can we do anything to improve the situation by perhaps implementing an approach with our students that could help to make the situation more wholesome?. More precisely, the question is, whether the North American Society for Sport Management and other sport management societies *can*, and indeed *should*, re-orient themselves to play a significant role in helping sport and physical activity become a *social institution* exerting a *positive influence* in the ongoing "adventure" of civilization.

To do this, sport management professional should determine what sort of a world he or she and descendants should be living in. If a person considers himself or herself to be an environmentalist, for example, the future looks bleak at present. If he/she is business oriented, however, the belief is that continued economic and technological growth could well be the answer to all upcoming problems. Finally, a person who is something of a "New Ager" can only hope for some sort of mass spiritual transformation will take place.

Homer-Dixon (2001), in his *The Ingenuity Gap*, believes that humans are changing their relationship with the world and are "careening into the future." He explains his belief that an "ingenuity gap" has been created, and he questions whether humans will be able to solve the environmental, technological, and social problems that have somehow developed. The searching question to all who are involved with sport management is in a similar vein. Will you have the necessary ingenuity to close the gap that has been created by the "commercialized sport juggernaut?" Will you live up to the highest purposes of any profession--that is, *to serve humankind best through the means at your disposal?*

Finally, it is probably the case that members of sport management societies are at the moment conforming blindly to the power structure as they use the medium of education and recreation--i.e., *sport*--for their selfish purposes. The author, as one aging person who encountered corruption and sleaze in the intercollegiate athletic structure of several major universities in the United States, retreated to a Canadian university where the term "scholar-athlete" still implied roughly what it says. However, serious problems are now developing in Canadian inter-university sport as well.

Two Approaches to Consider. What can this analysis possibly mean to members sport management worldwide? Actually there are several choices. One choice is to do nothing, meaning that NASSM, for example, continues in the same vein as at present. This would require no great effort. NASSM can simply continue to go along with the prevailing ethos of a society that is using sport to help promote more social, *as opposed to moral*, character traits. In the process, "business as usual" will be supported one way or the other-- by hook or by crook.

A second approach, recommended strongly, is that NASSM live up to the dictates of its constitution. Recall what Article II (Purpose) in the constitution calls for. After stating that NASSM should "promote, stimulate, and encourage study, research, scholarly writing, and professional development in the area of sport management *broadly interpreted* " [the italics are *not* the author's], it explains further that "this statement of purpose means that the members of this Society are concerned about the *theoretical* and *applied* aspects of management theory and practice specifically related to sport, exercise, dance, and play as these enterprises are pursued by all sectors of the population "

Still further, the constitution states that "in the furtherance of these aims and objectives, the Society shall endeavor to carry out the following functions: (1) support and cooperate with local, regional, national, and international organizations having similar purposes, (2) organize and administer meetings to promote the purpose stated above, and (3) issue appropriate proceedings and journals." It should not be necessary to press this point any further. At present the farthest thing from NASSM's "collective mind" would be to show steady, deliberative concern about the theoretical and applied aspects of management theory and practice *as related to exercise, dance, and play*. Who knows what the "body of knowledge" adds up to!

What NASSM's conference programs *are* showing deliberate concern about to a great extent--and doing it quite nicely--are the theoretical and applied aspects of commercialized sport management (i.e., management *quite narrowly interpreted*). This in itself is good, However, this is simply not enough for a professional society of high quality. And, to repeat, this is especially true if one reads the constitution. *What most NASSM members are doing, it is suggested, is devoting themselves to the type of sport that in the final analysis means least to our society and ignoring that which could mean the most!* NASSM should be seeking the answers to such questions as (1) what is sport's prevailing drift?; (2) what are the advantages and disadvantages of sport involvement for life?; and (3) what is sport's residual impact on society?

The author was personally involved in sport competitively throughout high school and college, and then coached university football, wrestlng, and/or swimming over a period of 15 years. Yet, he has personally been conducting an informal boycott of the NFL, NBA, and NFL, and of all *commercialized* university sport for years. Frankly, to him it has become disgusting, because it is basically non-educational and involves too much passive spectatoritis. It is actually subversive to the higher purposes of democracy.

Further, the author is convinced that the commercialized Olympic Movement with its drugs, officiating, free-loading officials and bribery problems, not to mention its millionaire basketball and hockey players, will eventually suffer the same fate as the ancient Games did *unless* radical change takes place. The late Baron de Coubertin and Avery Brundage must be "whirling in their graves" at a rate to soon exceed the sound barrier!

Concluding Statement

Is the author being unduly pessimistic, having reached the "old-curmudgeon" stage? Perhaps this is true. However, professionals in sport management societies, wherever you may be, are strongly urged to adhere--in both their research and professional actions--to their stated and approved purpose more carefully than they may be doing at present. In the immediate future, please seek the answer to two fundamental questions. The response to the first question might well cause action to be taken in the future to answer question #2. These questions are: (1) in what ways can we accurately assess the present status of sport to learn if it is--*or is not*--fulfilling its role as a presumably beneficent social institution? and (2)--depending on the answer to #1, of course--will you then have the motivation and professional zeal to do your utmost to help sport achieve what could well be its rightful place in society? *Sport and related physical activity--broadly interpreted--can indeed be a worthwhile social institution contributing to the wellbeing and health of people of all ages and conditions.* As they say, "don't be part of *the problem*, be part of *the solution!*"

References

Anderson, W. T. (1997). *The future of the self: Inventing the postmodern person.* NY: Tarcher/Putnam.

Berman, M. (2001) *The twilight of American culture,* NY: W.W. Norton.

Blinde, E. M. & McCallister, S. G. (1999). Women, disability, and sport and physical fitness activity: The intersection of gender and disability dynamics. *Research Quarterly for Sport and Exercise,* 70, 3, 303-312.

Booth, F. W., & Chakravarthy, M. V. (2002). Cost and consequences of sedentary living: New battleground for an old enemy. *Research Digest (PCPFS),* 3, 16, 1-8.

Borgman, A. (1993) Crossing the postmodern divide. Chicago: The Univ. of Chicago Press.

Cryderman, K. (2001). Sport's culture of adultery. *The Vancouver Sun* (Canada), August 21, C5.

Depauw, K. P. (1997). The (in)visibility of disability: Cultural contexts and "sporting bodies," *Quest,* 49, 416-430

Encarta World English Dictionary, The. (1999). NY: St. Martin's Press.

Feschuk, S. (2002). Night of the Olympic dead. *National Post* (Canada), Feb. 16, B10.

Hahm, C. H., Beller, J. M., & Stoll, S .K. (1989). *The Hahm-Beller Values Choice Inventory.* Moscow, ID: Center for Ethics, The Univ. of Idaho.

Homer-Dixon, T. (2001). *The ingenuity gap.* Toronto: Vintage Canada.

Huntington, S. P. (1998). *The Clash of Civilizations (and the Remaking of World Order.* NY: Touchstone.

Huxley, J. (1957). *New wine for new bottles.* NY: Harper & Row.

Kavussanu, M. & Roberts, G. C. (2001). Moral functioning in sport: An achievement goal perspective. *Journal of Sport and Exercise Psychology,* 23, 37-54

Long, W. (2001. Athletes losing faith in hard work. *The Vancouver Sun* (Canada), Jan. 31. E5.

Lumpkin, A., Stoll, S. K., & Beller, J. M. (1999). *Sport ethics: Applications for fair play* (2nd Ed.). St. Louis: McGraw-Hill.

Malina, R. M. (2001). Tracking of physical activity across the lifespan. *Research Digest (PCPFS)*, 3-14, 1-8.

Muller, H. J. (1952) *The uses of the past.* NY: Mentor.

Naipaul, V. S. (Oct 30, 1990). "Our Universal Civilization." The 1990 Winston Lecture, The Manhattan Institute, New York *Review of Books*, p. 20.

National Association for Sport and Physical Education. (2001). The coaches code of conduct. *Strategies, Nov.-Dec., 11.*

Naylor, D. (2002), In pursuit of level playing fields. *The Globe and Mail* (Canada), March 9, S1.

Priest, R. F., Krause, J. V., & Beach, J. (1999). Four-year changes in college athletes' ethical value choices in sports situations. *Research Quarterly for Exercise and Sport*, 70, 1, 170-178.

Province, The (Vancouver, Canada) (2000). Drug allegations rock sports world. July 3, A2.

Rudd, A., Stoll, S. K., & Beller, J. M. (1999). Measuring moral and social character among a group of Division 1A college athletes, non-athletes, and ROTC military students. *Research Quarterly for Exercise and Sport*, 70 (Suppl. 1), 127.

Sage, G. H. (1988, October). "Sports participation as a builder of character?" *The World and I*, Vol. 3, 629-641.

Schlesinger, A. M. (1998). (Rev. & Enl.).*The disuniting of America.* NY: W.W. Norton.

Skaset, H. B., Email correspondence. May 14, 2002.

Tibbetts, J. (2002). Spend more on popular sports, Canadians say, *National Post* (Canada), A8, April 15.

Toynbee, A. J. (1947). *A study of history.* NY: Oxford University Press.

Wallis, D. (2002). Annals of Olympics filled with dubious decisions. *National Post* (Canada), Feb. 16, B2.

Weiner, J. (Jan.-Feb. 2000). Why our obsession has ruined the game; and how we can save it.
Utne Reader, **97,** 48-50.

Zeigler, E. F. (1989). *An introduction to sport and physical education philosophy.* Carmel, IN: Benchmark.

Zeigler, E.F. (1996). Historical perspective on "quality of life": Genes, memes, and physical activity. *Quest* , 48, 246-263.